THE
DETOX
BLUEPRINT

*Ancient Wisdom and Modern Biology
for Lasting Detox.*

PeterJohn Fox

Disclaimer & Educational Use Statement

This book is intended for educational and informational purposes only.

The content within The Detox Blueprint is designed to help readers better understand general principles related to nutrition, lifestyle, detoxification systems, and overall wellness. It is not intended to diagnose, treat, cure, or prevent any disease, nor is it a substitute for professional medical advice, diagnosis, or treatment.

The information presented reflects a synthesis of traditional wellness perspectives, modern biological research, and educational interpretation. Individual needs, conditions, and responses can vary widely. What works well for one person may not be appropriate for another.

Readers should always consult with a qualified healthcare professional before making changes to diet, supplementation, exercise routines, or lifestyle practices—especially if they have a medical condition, are pregnant or nursing, are taking medications, or have concerns about their health.

Nothing in this book should be interpreted as medical advice or as a recommendation to discontinue prescribed treatments or medications without appropriate professional guidance.

The author and publisher assume no responsibility for any adverse effects or consequences resulting from the use or application of the information contained in this book.

By reading this book, you acknowledge that you are responsible for your own health decisions and that this material is provided as a general educational resource to support informed choices.

CONTENTS

Preface   i

Author's Note   v

1   Detox Isn't a Trend   1

2   What Toxins Really Are   9

3   The Liver - Your Master Detox Organ   18

4   The Gut, the Microbiome, and Elimination   27

5   Metabolic Stability, Blood Sugar, and Detox   35

6   Food as Information, Not Just Fuel   42

7   Building Detox-Supportive Meals That Work   49

8   Herbs, Roots, and Targeted Support   57

9   Movement, Circulation, and Sweat   64

10 Living the Blueprint   71

Afterword: From Understanding to Mastery   82

References   86

PREFACE

Most people come to the idea of detox because something feels off.

Energy feels inconsistent. Digestion feels unpredictable. Sleep no longer restores the way it used to. The body sends quiet signals long before it sends loud ones, and detox is often discovered in that in-between space - when you are not sick enough to be diagnosed, but not well enough to feel grounded.

This book was written for that space.

The Detox Blueprint is not about chasing symptoms or reacting to fear. It is about understanding how the body was designed to clear, balance, and recover when the right conditions are present. Detox, as presented here, is not an aggressive act. It is a cooperative one. When daily rhythms, nourishment, movement, and rest align, detox happens naturally, often without drama.

You may have already noticed that much of the confusion around detox comes from extremes. Some approaches promise rapid cleansing through restriction and intensity. Others dismiss detox altogether as unnecessary or mythical. The truth, as is often the case, lives between those poles. The body does detox. It does it constantly. What varies is how supported, or disrupted, that process becomes through modern life.

This book exists to bring clarity to that reality.

Throughout these chapters, you will find a blend of traditional wisdom and modern biology. Long before laboratory testing and metabolic pathways were named, cultures understood the importance of rhythm, simplicity, and seasonal balance. Today, science helps explain why those patterns worked. When these perspectives are held together rather than in opposition, detox stops being mysterious and starts becoming practical.

You will not find rigid rules here. You will find a framework.

A blueprint does not tell you exactly how to build every structure. It shows you how the pieces fit together so that your choices make sense. Food, movement, herbs, stress, sleep, and elimination are not separate topics - they are connected systems. When they work together, the body becomes more resilient and forgiving.

This book is meant to be educational first. It is designed to help you understand why certain approaches support detox, not just what to do. That understanding is what allows detox to move from a temporary phase into a sustainable way of living.

Alongside this book, there is a companion resource designed to help translate these ideas into daily practice: *the 15-Day Detox Planner.*

If you are already using the planner, consider this book the deeper context behind it. The planner gives structure to your days - meals, reflections, habits - while this book explains the systems those actions support. Together, they form a complete foundation.

If you have not yet accessed the planner, you will find a **link and QR code** included on the next page.

From there, you can download the **free PDF version** or choose to purchase a **printed copy** if you prefer something tangible to write in and return to. The planner is not required to benefit from this book, but it can greatly enhance how easily these concepts integrate into real life.

It is important to understand that detox is not a finish line. It is a relationship.

There will be seasons when your body needs more support and seasons when the foundation alone is enough. The goal is not constant intervention. The goal is awareness - knowing when to simplify, when to restore rhythm, and when to let the body do what it was designed to do.

This book does not replace medical care, nor does it attempt to diagnose or treat disease. It is an educational guide meant to help you make informed choices and to better understand how daily habits interact with the body's natural processes.

As you move through these chapters, read with curiosity rather than urgency. Let the ideas settle. Notice what resonates. Detox works best when it is approached with patience and respect, not pressure.

The blueprint is already there.

This book simply helps you see it... and learn how to live by it.

Scan the QR Code below
with the camera on your phone

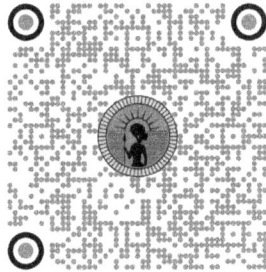

www.ancientafricansecrets.com/15-day-detox-planner-printed

AUTHOR'S NOTE

I did not set out to write a detox book because it was trendy.

I wrote this because, over time, I began to notice a pattern... both in my own life and in the lives of people around me. Many were doing "everything right" according to modern advice, yet still felt depleted, inflamed, disconnected from their bodies, or dependent on constant intervention just to feel normal. Health had become something outsourced, fragmented, and increasingly complicated.

That never sat right with me.

My worldview is rooted in the belief that the human body is intentionally designed - ordered, intelligent, and capable. Not fragile. Not random. Not in need of constant correction. When systems break down, it is rarely because the body has failed. More often, it is because the conditions it was designed to operate within have been quietly removed.

This belief is what led me to write Ancient African Secrets to Great Health.

That book was my attempt to reclaim something that had been largely ignored: the depth of traditional African wellness knowledge and its emphasis on food as medicine, rhythm as regulation, and lifestyle as the foundation of health. Across many African cultures, health was not treated as a series of isolated symptoms. It was understood as balance, between nourishment and movement, work and rest, environment and body.

What struck me most as I studied these traditions was how little contradiction existed between ancestral wisdom and modern biology when both were approached honestly. Where ancient cultures spoke of stagnation, modern science describes impaired circulation or lymphatic flow. Where tradition emphasized bitterness and plant diversity, research now highlights digestive signaling, bile flow, and detox enzyme activation.

The language differs, but the principles align.

This book is a continuation of that work.

The Detox Blueprint exists to bridge understanding, not to romanticize the past, and not to idolize modern science, but to let each inform the other. I believe truth is coherent. When something is real, it holds up across time, culture, and observation.

I do not approach health from the assumption that humans are accidental products of chaos. I approach it from the conviction that life has structure, purpose, and design. That conviction shapes how I interpret biology, metabolism, and healing. It is why I emphasize support over force, rhythm over extremes, and stewardship over control.

Detox, in this context, is not about purging or punishment. It is about restoration.

Over the years, I have watched detox become both overhyped and dismissed. Some turn it into an aggressive battle against the body. Others deny its relevance entirely. Both miss the point. The body detoxes every day. The real question is whether modern life is helping or hindering that process.

I wrote this book to answer that question clearly.

You will not find miracle claims here. You will not find fear-based language. You will not be told that your body is broken or toxic beyond repair. Instead, you will find education - grounded in physiology, informed by tradition, and shaped by lived observation.

This book is meant to restore confidence.

Confidence in the body's ability to adapt. Confidence in simple, repeatable habits. Confidence that health does not require constant complexity to be effective. When people understand why something works, they no longer need to be pushed. They choose wisely because it makes sense.

I am also aware that no book can replace wisdom gained through practice.

That is why this work is paired with tools like the 15-Day Detox Planner and, for those who want to go deeper, structured learning experiences beyond this book. Education should empower action, not create dependency.

Ultimately, my hope is simple.

That this book helps you reconnect with your body as something trustworthy rather than adversarial. That it encourages patience where there has been urgency, simplicity where there has been overwhelm, and responsibility where there has been confusion.

Health is not something we conquer.

It is something we cultivate.

If this book helps you take even one step toward living in greater alignment with how your body was designed to function, then it has done its job.

Peter John Fox

CHAPTER 1

Detox Isn't A Trend

For many people, the word detox immediately brings up images of extreme cleanses, rigid rules, and short bursts of discomfort that promise quick results. Over time, detox has been packaged as something dramatic: a temporary solution meant to undo months or years of overload in a matter of days. This framing has done more harm than good. It has confused people, discouraged consistency, and disconnected detox from the actual systems that make it possible.

But before the juice fasts, the thirty-day challenges, and the celebrity-endorsed protocols, there was something far quieter and far older. There was the body itself, doing what it has always done: clearing, filtering, renewing, and restoring balance without fanfare or force.

Detox did not begin as a trend. It describes a real and necessary biological process. Every day, your body produces waste as a natural result of living. Hormones are used and broken down. Cells generate byproducts as they produce energy. Foreign compounds enter through food, water, air, and skin. None of this is abnormal. The question is not whether waste exists, but whether the body is able to manage it efficiently.

This distinction matters more than most people realize. When we speak of detox as though it were something we do to the body, we miss the deeper truth: detox is something the body already does, constantly, without waiting for permission or a product.

The Body as a Self-Cleaning System

Consider for a moment how extraordinary the body's design actually is.

At this very second, your liver is receiving blood from two sources: the hepatic artery, carrying oxygen-rich blood from the heart, and the portal vein, carrying nutrient-laden blood from the digestive tract. Everything you ate today, every compound that crossed your intestinal lining, passed through the liver before reaching the rest of your body. This is not an accident. The liver is positioned as the body's first line of metabolic defense, and its filtering capacity is remarkable. In a healthy adult, the liver processes roughly 1.5 liters of blood per minute[44]. That means your entire blood volume passes through your liver multiple times each hour.

While the liver works, the kidneys are filtering plasma at a rate of approximately 120 milliliters per minute, extracting water-soluble waste and excess minerals before returning cleaned blood to circulation[13]. The lungs are expelling volatile compounds with every exhale. The skin is releasing certain substances through sweat. The gut is deciding what stays and what leaves, binding toxins to bile and fiber for elimination. The lymphatic system, often overlooked, is quietly transporting fluid and cellular debris toward processing stations where the immune system can evaluate threats.

This is not occasional activity. This is constant, coordinated labor happening every second of every day.

True detox is not about forcing toxins out of the body. It is about supporting the systems that already exist to handle them. When those systems are supported, detox happens quietly. When they are overwhelmed or under-resourced, symptoms appear.

Why Detox Became a Trend (and Why That's a Problem)

The modern detox industry did not emerge from nowhere. It grew out of a real and legitimate concern: that modern life places unprecedented demands on the body's natural clearing systems. This concern is valid. What followed, however, was often not.

Beginning in the late twentieth century, as public awareness of environmental pollution, food additives, and chemical exposure increased, a market opportunity appeared. Companies and wellness personalities began offering solutions to a problem that felt urgent and invisible. Detox became something you could buy: a program, a supplement stack, a restricted diet, a weekend retreat.

The problem was not the recognition that the body needed support. The problem was how that support was framed.

Instead of teaching people how detox actually works, the industry promoted urgency and fear. Instead of emphasizing steady, sustainable habits, it promoted extremes: aggressive cleanses, severe restriction, and dramatic interventions that promised rapid results. The body, which had been clearing waste for millennia without instruction manuals, was suddenly portrayed as incapable of functioning without intervention.

This approach backfired in several important ways.

First, extreme restriction often impairs detox rather than enhancing it. The liver relies on a steady supply of nutrients to perform its work. The binding processes that neutralize and prepare toxins for elimination require amino acids, B vitamins, magnesium, selenium, and other compounds that come from food[20]. When caloric intake drops too low, or when entire macronutrient groups are eliminated, the liver loses access to raw materials. Research shows that severe caloric restriction can reduce liver enzyme activity and slow metabolic processes rather than accelerate them[1]. In practical terms, the person trying to "detox harder" is often making it harder for their liver to do its job.

Second, extreme approaches often release stored toxins faster than the body can process them. Many environmental compounds are fat-soluble, meaning they dissolve in fat rather than water. The body stores these compounds in adipose tissue as a protective mechanism, keeping them away from vital organs. This storage is not failure; it is intelligent design. The problem arises when fat tissue releases these compounds faster than the liver and gut can handle them. This often happens during rapid weight loss, aggressive fasting, or high-stress detox protocols. Research confirms that adipose tissue acts as a reservoir for persistent organic pollutants and that rapid mobilization of fat stores can increase circulating toxin levels[26]. The result is often increased symptoms, not relief.

Third, the drama of extreme detox discouraged consistency. When detox is framed as a painful, short-term ordeal, most people cannot sustain it. They push through a few days or weeks, experience discomfort, and then return to old habits. The cycle repeats: burden, crisis intervention, burden, crisis intervention. Meanwhile, the steady, unglamorous work of supporting daily detox goes unaddressed.

This pattern has created widespread confusion. People now associate detox with discomfort rather than ease. They believe that feeling worse is a sign of progress. They chase intensity when what the body actually needs is stability.

What Detox Actually Looks Like

Your body is detoxing all the time. This is not something it turns on and off. The liver is constantly transforming waste into safer forms. The kidneys are filtering the blood. The digestive tract is deciding what leaves and what stays. The lungs remove volatile compounds, while the skin and lymphatic system assist in transport and elimination. Detox is not an event. It is a continuous, coordinated effort.

Understanding this continuity changes everything about how detox should be approached.

When detox pathways are working well, you rarely notice them. Energy is steady. Digestion is predictable. Sleep is restorative. The mind is clear. The body moves through its days without accumulating the kind of burden that eventually demands attention.

When detox pathways are not working well, the body sends signals. Fatigue, headaches, bloating, brain fog, skin changes, and mood shifts are often signs that detox systems are struggling to keep up. These symptoms are not failures. They are messages. They indicate that something in the balance between input and output has shifted, and that the body is asking for support.

This is where modern detox approaches often go wrong. Instead of listening to these signals and lowering the burden, many programs push the body harder. More supplements. Longer fasts. Greater restriction. More sweat. The assumption is that intensity produces results.

But intensity without support often produces strain.

A more effective approach is support rather than acceleration. Detox works best when the body has what it needs and is not being constantly challenged. This means adequate hydration to support transport. It means sufficient protein to support binding. It means fiber to support elimination. It means rest to support repair. It means reducing the inputs that create unnecessary burden while providing the nutrients that make clearance possible.

This is not dramatic. It is not impressive on social media. But it is how the body was designed to function.

Traditional Wisdom and Modern Biology

Long before modern science named detox pathways, traditional wellness systems understood something important: the body clears best when life is steady, simple, and rhythmic.

In many African traditions, detox was not treated as a dramatic intervention. It was built into daily life. Meals were simple and repetitive, reducing the constant metabolic decision-making that modern diets demand. Bitter plants were used regularly, not as emergency measures, but as ongoing support for digestion and elimination. Movement was constant, not because anyone called it "exercise," but because life itself required walking, carrying, bending, and working. Rest followed labor. Seasons dictated rhythms. The body was not seen as something to fix, but as something to cooperate with.

Modern research increasingly validates what traditional systems practiced through experience.

Bitter foods, for example, were valued not for taste alone, but for their effect on digestion and elimination. Today, research confirms that bitter compounds influence digestive secretions and liver-related processes. Bitter taste receptors exist not only in the mouth but throughout the gastrointestinal tract, and activation of these receptors influences gut hormones, bile flow, and metabolic signaling[10]. When traditional cultures ate bitter greens, roots, and herbs as part of regular meals, they were quietly supporting the same pathways that modern supplements attempt to target.

Fiber-rich plant foods supported regular elimination, ensuring that waste bound to bile actually left the body rather than being reabsorbed. Research on enterohepatic circulation shows that when digestion is sluggish, hormone metabolites and other waste compounds can be recycled back into the bloodstream instead of eliminated[36]. Traditional diets, built around whole plants and roots, kept this exit route functioning.

Naturally fermented foods helped maintain balance in the gut microbiome, which plays a central role in how effectively the body handles waste. Modern studies confirm that gut bacteria directly influence how bile acids, hormones, and foreign compounds are processed in the intestines[8].

Movement supported lymphatic flow, which does not have its own pump and depends on physical activity to move fluid[16]. Traditional life, with its constant low-level physical demands, kept lymph moving without requiring dedicated "exercise sessions."

Sweating, whether from labor or heat, provided an additional exit route for certain compounds. Research shows that some metals and fat-soluble substances can be excreted through sweat, although this pathway is secondary to liver and gut elimination[39].

These practices worked not because they were extreme, but because they were consistent. They did not overwhelm the body. They supported flow.

The Modern Challenge

The challenge today is not that the body has changed, but that the environment has. Modern life introduces a level of chemical, dietary, and psychological load that previous generations did not face.

Consider what the average person encounters in a single day. Processed foods containing dozens of additives and synthetic compounds. Water treated with chemicals and carried through aging infrastructure. Air filled with particulate matter, vehicle emissions, and off-gassed compounds from building materials. Personal care products containing preservatives, fragrances, and stabilizers. Household cleaners, plastics, synthetic fabrics, and electronic devices all contribute their own signatures.

None of these factors are necessarily catastrophic on their own, but together they create cumulative burden.

Cumulative burden matters more than any single exposure. When the total load exceeds the body's ability to eliminate waste efficiently, detox slows down. The liver prioritizes immediate survival needs over long-term cleanup. The gut becomes inflamed or sluggish. The lymphatic system stagnates. Fat tissue stores compounds that cannot be processed right away.

Research shows that repeated low-level exposure can place chronic stress on detox systems even when individual exposures fall below levels considered immediately harmful[17]. This is one reason people can feel unwell without a single clear cause. The problem is not one toxin. The problem is the total.

Add to this the psychological dimension of modern life: chronic stress, fragmented sleep, constant stimulation, and the kind of low-grade anxiety that never quite resolves. Stress hormones themselves require processing and elimination. When the nervous system stays activated, digestive function decreases, inflammation increases, and detox becomes harder[7].

This understanding reframes detox entirely. The aim is not to eliminate every possible exposure or achieve a state of purity. The aim is to lower background stress so the body can regain efficiency. Small, consistent reductions in burden often produce better results than aggressive short-term interventions.

The Blueprint Approach

This book is built on that principle. The Detox Blueprint is not a medical manual or a quick-fix program. It does not diagnose conditions or replace professional care. Instead, it explains how detox works so you can make informed, grounded decisions.

The goal is not perfection. It is awareness and support.

Throughout this book, you will learn how detox systems function, why certain foods and habits help or hinder them, and how to work with your body instead of against it. You will also learn why many popular detox ideas fail: not because detox is flawed, but because the approach is misaligned with how the body was designed to function.

A blueprint does not tell you exactly how to build every structure. It shows you how the pieces fit together so that your choices make sense. Food, movement, herbs, stress, sleep, and elimination are not separate topics. They are connected systems. When they work together, the body becomes more resilient and forgiving.

The *15-Day Detox Planner* you may have already completed was intentionally simple. It focused on hydration, gentle meals, movement, rest, and reflection. It showed you what to do. This book explains why those actions work and how to turn them into lasting habits.

There is no need to rush. Detox is not a race. It is a relationship with your body that improves over time.

With this foundation in place, the next step is to understand what the body is actually dealing with. In the next chapter, we will clarify what toxins truly are, where they come from, and why understanding toxic load matters more than fear or avoidance.

Detox begins with understanding. From there, everything becomes simpler.

CHAPTER 2

What Toxins Really Are

For many people, the word toxin carries an emotional charge. It suggests danger, contamination, and the sense that the modern world is somehow poisoning the body from all sides. Because of this, conversations about toxins often drift toward fear rather than understanding. But fear is not a helpful starting point. Clarity is.

The word itself has been stretched so far that it has almost lost meaning. In marketing, "toxin" often refers to anything a company wants you to avoid in order to sell you something else. In casual conversation, it sometimes becomes a vague stand-in for anything unpleasant: bad relationships, negative thoughts, or foods that someone simply dislikes. This looseness has made it harder for people to understand what the body is actually dealing with.

A toxin, in simple terms, is any substance that interferes with normal biological function when it accumulates beyond what the body can handle. That definition matters because it immediately removes the idea that toxins are rare, mysterious, or always external. Some toxins come from the environment. Others are produced inside the body every single day as a normal result of metabolism.

This is the first and most important distinction: toxicity is not about the substance alone. It is about the relationship between the substance, the dose, and the body's capacity to process it. Water, essential for life, becomes toxic if consumed in extreme excess. Oxygen, which every cell requires, generates reactive byproducts that the body must neutralize constantly. Even the hormones that regulate mood, metabolism, and reproduction become problematic if they are not cleared after completing their work.

Understanding toxins clearly is the foundation of understanding detox. When the conversation moves from fear to biology, everything becomes more practical.

The Body Produces Waste Every Day

Life itself produces waste. This is not a flaw in the design. It is simply how biological systems work.

Every time cells generate energy, byproducts are created. The mitochondria, often called the powerhouses of the cell, convert nutrients into usable energy through a process that inevitably produces reactive oxygen species. These molecules are chemically unstable, and if left unchecked, they can damage cellular structures. The body manages this through antioxidant systems that neutralize reactive oxygen before it causes harm. Under healthy conditions, this process runs smoothly. Under stress, illness, or nutrient deficiency, the balance can shift[14].

Protein metabolism generates its own set of byproducts. When proteins are broken down for energy or recycled for repair, the nitrogen they contain must be removed. The body converts this nitrogen into ammonia, a compound that is toxic to the brain and nervous system even in small amounts. The liver rapidly transforms ammonia into urea, a much safer compound that the kidneys can then filter into urine. This conversion happens constantly, quietly, without any conscious awareness. In a healthy adult, the liver processes and converts ammonia around the clock, preventing accumulation that would otherwise cause confusion, lethargy, and eventually coma[19].

Hormones are another source of internal waste that rarely enters the detox conversation. People tend to think of hormones only in terms of production: whether the body is making enough estrogen, testosterone, thyroid hormone, or cortisol. But hormones are designed to act briefly and then be deactivated and removed. A hormone that lingers beyond its signaling window can create imbalance even when production itself is normal.

Estrogen offers a clear example. After estrogen completes its work, the liver transforms it into metabolites that can be excreted through bile and urine. Some of these metabolites are relatively harmless. Others are more reactive and potentially problematic if they accumulate. The pathway the liver uses to process estrogen, and how quickly the gut eliminates the metabolites, directly influences hormonal balance. Research shows that variations in estrogen metabolism are associated with differences in health outcomes, particularly for hormonally sensitive tissues[38].

Cellular turnover adds another layer. The body is constantly replacing old cells with new ones. Red blood cells, for instance, live for roughly 120 days before being broken down and recycled. The hemoglobin they contain is processed into bilirubin, a yellow pigment that gives bruises their characteristic color as they heal. The liver conjugates bilirubin and excretes it through bile. When this process is impaired, bilirubin accumulates in the blood and tissues, producing the yellowing of skin and eyes known as jaundice.

None of this internal waste production is abnormal. It is a sign of life, not dysfunction. The question is never whether the body produces waste. The question is whether elimination keeps pace with production.

External Sources of Toxic Load

While the body has always dealt with internal waste, modern life has added an entirely new dimension to the equation. Humans have always encountered substances in the environment, but the scale and variety of those encounters have changed dramatically over the past century.

The chemical revolution of the twentieth century transformed nearly every aspect of daily life. Plastics, pesticides, pharmaceuticals, preservatives, flame retardants, industrial solvents, and synthetic fragrances entered commerce faster than their long-term effects could be studied. By some estimates, more than 80,000 synthetic chemicals are now in commercial use, and only a small fraction have been thoroughly tested for human health effects[27]. This is not a conspiracy. It is simply the pace at which industrial innovation outran regulatory science.

The result is that the average person now encounters compounds their great-grandparents never knew existed. Phthalates from plastics. Bisphenols from food packaging. Parabens from personal care products. Glyphosate from agricultural herbicides. Perfluorinated compounds from nonstick cookware and water-resistant fabrics. Heavy metals from industrial emissions, older infrastructure, and certain foods. The list continues.

Many of these substances are not acutely poisonous in the amounts typically encountered. A single exposure to a small quantity of any one compound is unlikely to cause immediate harm. Their impact comes from repetition and accumulation. Day after day, year after year, small exposures add up. Scientific research shows that repeated low-level exposure can place chronic stress on detox systems even when individual exposures fall below levels considered immediately harmful[17].

This distinction between acute toxicity and chronic burden is essential. Much of the confusion around environmental health comes from conflating these two concepts. A substance can be safe in a single dose but problematic when encountered continuously. A substance can pass regulatory tests for acute toxicity while still contributing to long-term metabolic strain. The dose makes the poison, as the old saying goes, but so does the duration.

Diet and Daily Habits

Diet plays a central role in determining toxic load, and not only because of what might be "in" the food. The quality and composition of what a person eats influences how well the body can handle everything else.

Ultra-processed foods introduce their own set of compounds the body must neutralize. Artificial colors, synthetic preservatives, flavor enhancers, emulsifiers, and texturizers are all biologically active substances that require processing. At the same time, these foods often displace nutrient-dense options that would otherwise support detox pathways. The liver needs amino acids, B vitamins, magnesium, zinc, and other nutrients to perform its binding and elimination work. A diet dominated by processed foods tends to increase burden while decreasing support.

Studies consistently link diets high in ultra-processed foods with increased markers of oxidative stress and inflammation[33]. Oxidative stress and inflammation both interfere with detox efficiency. They consume resources that would otherwise be available for clearance. They create additional byproducts that require processing. They shift the body toward a state of low-grade chronic burden rather than efficient maintenance.

Alcohol deserves specific mention. Unlike most dietary components, alcohol is directly toxic to cells and must be prioritized for clearance. When alcohol enters the body, the liver shifts resources toward processing it, temporarily deprioritizing other detox functions. The metabolic byproduct of alcohol breakdown, acetaldehyde, is itself more toxic than the original alcohol and must be quickly converted to a safer form. Frequent or heavy alcohol consumption places ongoing demand on the liver's detox capacity, leaving less room for everything else.

Excess sugar, particularly fructose consumed in large amounts, adds metabolic stress of a different kind. Unlike glucose, which can be used by cells throughout the body, fructose is processed almost exclusively by the liver. High fructose intake has been associated with increased liver fat accumulation, oxidative stress, and impaired metabolic function[23]. A liver burdened by excessive fructose metabolism has fewer resources for its other detoxification roles.

Industrial seed oils, consumed in quantities unheard of a century ago, introduce highly oxidizable fatty acids into the body. When these fats oxidize, they generate compounds that require antioxidant and detox resources to neutralize. While the debate over specific oils continues, the broader point is straightforward: the modern diet contains fats that oxidize more readily than traditional fats, adding another dimension to overall burden[11].

Hormones, Medications, and Overlapping Systems

The detox equation becomes more complex when hormones and medications enter the picture.

Hormones, as mentioned earlier, must be cleared after they complete their signaling work. The liver plays a central role in hormone metabolism, while the digestive tract determines whether hormone byproducts leave the body or are reabsorbed. Research on enterohepatic circulation shows that when gut transit is slow, hormone metabolites that were packaged for elimination can be recycled back into circulation instead[36]. This explains why detox, digestion, and hormonal balance are inseparable. A sluggish gut can create hormonal imbalance even when hormone production itself is normal.

Environmental compounds can complicate this further. Many synthetic chemicals are structurally similar enough to hormones that they can interact with hormone receptors, either mimicking or blocking normal signaling. These are often called endocrine-disrupting compounds. Bisphenol A, certain phthalates, and some pesticides fall into this category. Research shows that low-dose exposures to combinations of these compounds can disrupt hormonal signaling even when each substance alone appears harmless[24]. The body must not only clear its own hormones but also manage the interference from hormone-mimicking compounds in the environment.

Medications add another dimension. Pharmaceuticals can be essential and life-saving, and this book is not anti-medicine. At the same time, medications are biologically active compounds that must be metabolized and cleared. Drug metabolism relies heavily on liver enzyme systems, particularly the cytochrome P450 family, that also process environmental toxins, hormones, and dietary compounds[47].

When multiple medications are taken simultaneously, or when medications are combined with alcohol, certain supplements, or specific foods, competition for these enzyme systems can occur. One substance may be processed more slowly because another substance is occupying the same pathway. This is the basis of many drug interactions. It is also a reminder that the liver's detox capacity is not infinite. Every compound that requires processing draws from the same pool of resources.

Awareness of these interactions is not meant to create fear of medication. It is meant to create understanding. When someone is taking multiple pharmaceuticals, supporting overall detox capacity through diet, hydration, and lifestyle becomes even more important, not less.

The Concept of Total Load

One of the most important ideas in modern toxicology is that total load matters more than any single exposure. The body does not experience toxins in isolation. It experiences combinations.

Consider a typical morning. A person wakes up and showers using products that contain synthetic fragrances and preservatives. They dry off with a towel washed in detergent with optical brighteners and fabric softeners. They apply deodorant, lotion, and perhaps cosmetics, each with its own ingredient list. They drink coffee that may contain trace pesticide residues, eat food that may include additives, and breathe air that carries particles from traffic, cleaning products, and building materials. They check their phone, which off-gasses small amounts of flame retardants. They drive to work in a vehicle with synthetic interior materials.

None of these individual exposures is likely to cause immediate harm. But the total, accumulated across a day, a week, a year, and a lifetime, becomes significant. The liver and kidneys do not process these compounds one at a time in neat sequence. They process them simultaneously, prioritizing, competing, and adapting as best they can.

This understanding reframes detox entirely. Detox is not about identifying a single villain. It is about reducing overall burden so the body's systems can function efficiently again.

The concept of total load also explains why two people can have such different responses to similar exposures. One person seems unbothered by a lifestyle that leaves another person exhausted, inflamed, and symptomatic. The difference often lies in their starting capacity: the efficiency of their detox enzymes (which has genetic variation), the state of their gut health, their nutritional status, their stress levels, and how much burden they were already carrying before the latest exposure arrived.

Reducing total load is almost always more effective than obsessing over any single compound. Lowering the overall burden on detox systems allows the body to process what remains more efficiently.

Fat Tissue and Long-Term Storage

Fat tissue plays a unique role in the toxin story, one that is often misunderstood.

Many environmental compounds are fat-soluble, meaning they dissolve in fat rather than water. When these compounds enter the body faster than the liver can process them, the body stores them in adipose tissue as a protective mechanism. This keeps them away from vital organs like the brain, heart, and kidneys. Storage is not failure. It is intelligent triage.

Research confirms that adipose tissue acts as a reservoir for persistent organic pollutants, including certain pesticides, flame retardants, and industrial chemicals[26]. These compounds can remain stored for years, slowly releasing over time as fat tissue turns over.

While this storage reduces immediate harm, it creates a long-term challenge. Stored compounds are not gone. They are waiting. During periods of stress, illness, or rapid weight loss, fat tissue breaks down more quickly, releasing stored compounds back into circulation. If the liver and gut are not prepared for this release, symptoms can increase rather than decrease.

This is one reason aggressive detox strategies often backfire. Rapid fat loss through extreme caloric restriction or intense exercise can mobilize stored toxins faster than the body can clear them. The person feels worse, not better, and often concludes that detox does not work or that they must push even harder. In reality, the pace was simply faster than their clearance capacity could handle.

The wiser approach is gradual. When fat loss occurs slowly and elimination pathways are well supported, stored compounds release at a rate the body can manage. Detox becomes steady rather than dramatic.

Moving from Fear to Strategy

Understanding toxins clearly changes the goal of detox. The aim is not to eliminate every possible exposure or achieve a state of purity. Purity is neither possible nor necessary. The aim is to lower background stress, support elimination pathways, and restore balance.

When the conversation moves from fear to strategy, practical choices become clearer. Reducing obvious sources of burden, like ultra-processed foods, excessive alcohol, and unnecessary chemical exposures in personal care and household products, lowers total load. Supporting detox capacity through adequate nutrition, hydration, fiber, and rest gives the body what it needs to do its work. Maintaining steady metabolic and digestive function ensures that waste actually leaves rather than being recycled.

None of this requires perfection. It requires direction. Small, consistent changes in the right direction often produce greater benefit than extreme short-term interventions.

With a clear understanding of what toxins are and where they come from, the next step is to explore how the body manages this load. In the next chapter, we turn our focus to the liver, the central organ responsible for transforming toxins and preparing them for safe removal.

Understanding toxic load removes fear. From that place, detox becomes practical, sustainable, and effective.

CHAPTER 3

The Liver - Your Master Detox Organ

If detox had a center of gravity, it would be the liver. Quietly and constantly, it sits at the intersection of everything that enters the body and everything that must eventually leave. Food, drink, medications, hormones, and environmental compounds all pass through the liver in some form. Long before the body decides what to use, store, transform, or eliminate, the liver is already at work.

Because its work is mostly invisible, the liver is easy to overlook. Many people only think about it when something goes wrong. Yet detox depends on the liver every single day, not as a dramatic event, but as a steady background process that keeps internal balance intact.

Understanding how the liver works changes how you approach detox. It reveals why extreme interventions often backfire, why certain nutrients matter so much, and why patience consistently outperforms intensity.

An Extraordinary Organ

The liver is the largest internal organ in the human body, weighing roughly three pounds in an adult. It sits in the upper right portion of the abdomen, protected by the rib cage, and receives blood from two distinct sources. The hepatic artery delivers oxygen-rich blood from the heart. The portal vein delivers nutrient-rich blood directly from the digestive tract. This dual blood supply is not accidental. It reflects the liver's unique position as both a metabolic hub and a filtering station.

Everything absorbed from your intestines, whether nutrients, medications, or unwanted compounds, passes through the liver before reaching general circulation. This arrangement, known as first-pass metabolism, allows the liver to intercept and process substances before they can affect the rest of the body. It is an elegant design that places the body's most sophisticated chemical processing plant directly in the path of incoming material[44].

The liver performs over 500 distinct functions. It regulates blood sugar by storing and releasing glucose as needed. It produces bile, which is essential for fat digestion and waste elimination. It synthesizes proteins, including those that allow blood to clot. It stores vitamins and minerals. It converts ammonia, a toxic byproduct of protein metabolism, into urea for safe excretion. And it transforms countless foreign and internal compounds into forms the body can eliminate.

Perhaps most remarkably, the liver can regenerate. If a portion is removed or damaged, the remaining tissue can regrow to restore function. This regenerative capacity is nearly unique among human organs and speaks to the liver's importance. The body has invested heavily in ensuring this organ can recover from insult[32].

Yet regeneration has limits. Chronic overload, whether from alcohol, medications, environmental toxins, or metabolic stress, can eventually overwhelm the liver's ability to keep up. The goal of supporting detox is not to push the liver harder. It is to reduce the burden so the liver can work efficiently within its design.

How the Liver Transforms Toxins

One of the most persistent myths about detox is the idea that toxins are stored and then suddenly flushed out. The liver does not function like a drain. It does not dump toxins. Its role is far more careful and far more intelligent than that. The liver transforms substances so they can be safely handled by the rest of the body.

This transformation happens in stages. Scientists often describe these stages as Phase I and Phase II detoxification. These labels are not meant to complicate things. They simply describe the order in which the liver does its work.

In Phase I, the liver modifies compounds to prepare them for elimination.

Many toxins, whether produced internally or encountered externally, are fat-soluble. Fat-soluble substances cannot be easily excreted in urine or bile because they do not dissolve in water. The liver must first alter their chemical structure to make them more water-soluble and easier to eliminate.

Phase I relies primarily on a family of enzymes known as cytochrome P450. These enzymes are remarkably versatile, capable of processing thousands of different compounds. They work by adding or exposing reactive chemical groups on target molecules, essentially creating a "handle" that Phase II enzymes can grab onto[47].

There is an important nuance here that is often missed. During Phase I processing, some substances become temporarily more reactive. They are easier to process, but also more irritating if they remain in circulation too long. These intermediate metabolites can cause oxidative stress and cellular damage if they are not quickly moved along to Phase II. This is not a flaw in the design. It is simply how the chemistry works.

Phase II is where these reactive intermediates are neutralized. The liver attaches, or conjugates, these compounds to other molecules that render them harmless and water-soluble. Common conjugation pathways include glucuronidation, sulfation, glutathione conjugation, and amino acid conjugation. Each pathway has its own enzyme systems and its own nutrient requirements[18].

Once a compound has been conjugated, it can be safely transported to the kidneys for excretion in urine or to the intestines for excretion in bile and stool. The transformation is complete. What was once a potentially harmful fat-soluble substance is now a water-soluble, neutralized compound ready to leave the body.

When the Phases Fall Out of Balance

The relationship between Phase I and Phase II explains a great deal about why some people feel worse during detox attempts.

Problems arise when Phase I speeds up without adequate support for Phase II. Aggressive cleanses, extreme caloric restriction, certain supplements, and even some medications can accelerate Phase I activity. If Phase II cannot keep pace, partially processed compounds accumulate. These reactive intermediates circulate longer than they should, creating oxidative stress rather than relieving burden.

The symptoms are familiar to anyone who has pushed too hard during a cleanse: headaches, fatigue, skin flare-ups, irritability, brain fog, and general malaise. These are not signs that toxins are "leaving." More often, they are signs that the process is out of balance. Phase I has created intermediates that Phase II cannot clear quickly enough.

This understanding reframes the entire detox experience. Feeling worse is not evidence of success. In most cases, it is evidence of strain. Detox works best when both phases are supported and working in harmony.

Genetic variation adds another layer. People differ in the activity levels of their Phase I and Phase II enzymes. Some individuals have highly active Phase I systems but slower Phase II pathways. These people tend to be particularly sensitive to environmental exposures and may feel unwell in situations that others tolerate easily. Others have the opposite pattern. Understanding that these variations exist helps explain why detox experiences differ so much from person to person[29].

The Nutrients That Make Detox Possible

Both phases of liver detoxification depend heavily on nutrition. The liver cannot perform its work without raw materials. When those materials are missing, detox slows regardless of how many cleanses are attempted.

Phase I enzymes require B vitamins, particularly B2, B3, B6, B12, and folate. They also require minerals like magnesium, iron, and zinc. Adequate protein intake matters because amino acids serve as building blocks for enzyme production. When any of these nutrients are deficient, Phase I activity decreases[20].

Phase II has even more specific requirements. Glutathione conjugation, one of the most important Phase II pathways, depends on adequate glutathione levels. Glutathione is synthesized from three amino acids: cysteine, glycine, and glutamate. Cysteine is often the limiting factor, which is why sulfur-containing foods like eggs, garlic, onions, and cruciferous vegetables are frequently emphasized in detox-supportive diets.

Glucuronidation requires adequate glucose and B vitamins. Sulfation requires sulfur-containing amino acids and adequate sulfate. Amino acid conjugation requires glycine and taurine. Methylation, another important detox pathway, requires folate, B12, and methionine. Each pathway draws from the body's nutrient stores[29].

This explains why severe caloric restriction often impairs detox rather than supporting it. When food intake drops too low, the liver loses access to the very nutrients it needs to do its work. The person attempting to "cleanse" by eating less may actually be slowing their liver's processing capacity.

It also explains why nutrient-dense whole foods are so central to detox. A diet rich in vegetables, adequate protein, healthy fats, and diverse plant compounds provides the raw materials the liver needs. Supplements can help address specific deficiencies, but they work best when built on a foundation of real food.

Bile: The Liver's Exit Route

The liver's work does not end with transformation. Once compounds have been conjugated and neutralized, they must actually leave the body. This is where bile becomes essential.

Bile is a yellow-green fluid produced by the liver and stored in the gallbladder. Most people think of bile only in terms of fat digestion. When you eat a meal containing fat, the gallbladder contracts and releases bile into the small intestine, where it emulsifies fats and allows them to be absorbed. This digestive function is important, but it is only part of the story.

Bile is also a major vehicle for waste elimination. Many of the conjugated compounds produced by Phase II are excreted into bile and carried to the intestines. From there, they are meant to leave the body through stool. Fat-soluble toxins, spent hormones, cholesterol, and bilirubin all exit primarily through this bile-to-gut pathway[21].

When bile flow is sluggish, or when intestinal transit is slow, problems can arise. Some compounds that were packaged for elimination can be reabsorbed back into circulation through a process called enterohepatic circulation. Instead of leaving, they return to the liver, which must process them again. This recycling increases the liver's workload and can contribute to symptoms of burden even when the liver itself is functioning well.

Supporting bile flow becomes an important piece of the detox puzzle. Adequate fat in the diet stimulates bile release. Bitter foods and herbs have traditionally been used to support bile production and flow. Fiber in the intestines binds bile and the toxins it carries, helping ensure they leave the body rather than being recycled.

Traditional Wisdom and Modern Understanding

Traditional African wellness practices reflected an intuitive understanding of liver support long before modern biochemistry described it in scientific terms.

Bitter plants and roots were commonly used to stimulate digestion and support what we now understand as bile flow. Across many African cultures, bitterness was not avoided but embraced as medicine. Bitter leaves, roots, and barks were consumed regularly, not during special "detox" periods, but as part of normal eating. Modern research confirms that bitter compounds activate receptors throughout the digestive tract, influencing gastric secretions, gut hormones, and bile-related activity[31].

Meals were often simple and repetitive, reducing the variety of compounds the liver needed to process at any given time. This simplicity was not poverty of diet. It was metabolic wisdom. When the liver encounters the same familiar foods day after day, it can process them more efficiently. Novel compounds, additives, and unfamiliar substances require more adaptive effort.

Fermented foods, common in many traditional African diets, supported gut health and regular elimination. A healthy gut ensures that bile-bound waste actually leaves the body rather than being recycled. The connection between gut function and liver health, now well established in scientific literature, was practiced intuitively for generations.

Movement was built into daily life, not as exercise, but as living. Walking, carrying, working in fields, and tending to daily tasks kept circulation strong and supported the flow of blood through the liver. Sedentary living, by contrast, slows circulation and can contribute to sluggish hepatic function.

Rest followed labor in natural rhythm. The liver does significant repair and processing work during sleep, particularly during the deeper stages. Traditional patterns of early rising and early rest aligned with circadian rhythms that support liver function[35].

These practices worked not because they were extreme, but because they were consistent. They reduced burden while providing support. They worked with the body rather than against it.

Signs the Liver Is Asking for Support

The liver rarely sends dramatic signals until something is seriously wrong. Liver disease can progress silently for years. But the body does send subtle signs when detox capacity is strained, even if the liver itself remains technically healthy.

Persistent fatigue, especially fatigue that does not improve with rest, can indicate that the body is spending excessive energy on processing burden rather than on daily function. Sluggish digestion, bloating, and discomfort after fatty meals may suggest that bile flow is not optimal. Skin issues, including acne, rashes, and dull complexion, sometimes reflect the skin picking up elimination work that the liver and gut are not completing.

Poor tolerance to alcohol, medications, or strong smells can indicate that Phase I and Phase II are struggling to keep pace. Hormonal imbalances, particularly estrogen-related symptoms, may point to impaired hormone clearance through the liver. Mood changes, brain fog, and difficulty concentrating can occur when the liver is not efficiently clearing compounds that affect the nervous system.

These signs are not diagnoses. They are invitations to pay attention. They suggest that the balance between burden and capacity has shifted and that support may be needed.

Supporting the Liver Through Consistency

The liver responds best to consistency rather than intensity. Extreme interventions tend to work against the very goals they aim to achieve. Steady, sustainable support creates conditions where the liver can work efficiently day after day.

Regular hydration improves transport and helps the kidneys share the elimination workload. Adequate protein ensures the liver has amino acids for both Phase I and Phase II processes. Fiber supports bile binding and elimination through the gut. Colorful vegetables provide antioxidants that help manage the reactive intermediates produced during Phase I.

Reducing obvious sources of burden makes a meaningful difference. Limiting alcohol reduces one of the liver's most demanding processing tasks. Reducing ultra-processed foods lowers the intake of additives and synthetic compounds. Choosing cleaner personal care and household products decreases the environmental load the liver must handle.

Sleep matters more than most people realize. The liver follows circadian rhythms, and much of its repair and intensive processing occurs during sleep. Chronic sleep deprivation impairs liver function and reduces detox capacity[35]. Prioritizing rest is not indulgence. It is support.

The liver works best when the body feels safe, nourished, and stable. Detox is most effective when it fits into daily life rather than disrupting it.

With a clear understanding of the liver's role, the next piece of the detox puzzle becomes visible. Preparing waste is only half the process. Waste must actually leave the body. In the next chapter, we turn our attention to elimination, especially through the gut, and explore why detox often fails not because the liver is weak, but because waste has nowhere to go.

When the liver is supported and elimination is clear, detox becomes something the body does naturally, quietly, and effectively.

CHAPTER 4

The Gut, the Microbiome, and Elimination

Once the liver has done its work, detox is only halfway complete. Preparing waste is important, but preparation alone does not clear the burden. For detox to actually succeed, waste must leave the body. This is where many detox efforts quietly fail. Not because the liver is weak or broken, but because elimination is slow, incomplete, or overlooked entirely.

Think of it like taking out the trash. You can bag everything up perfectly, tie it neatly, and set it by the door. But if no one ever carries it outside, the trash is still in your house. It sits there, and eventually it starts causing problems.

The gut is where waste either leaves the body or gets stuck. It is the final checkpoint. And what happens there determines whether the liver's hard work actually pays off.

Detox Works Like a Relay

Detox is not a single action. It works more like a relay race, where different systems hand off responsibility to one another. The liver transforms compounds into safer forms, packages them up, and passes them along. But other systems must carry those packages the rest of the way out.

The gut plays the biggest role in this handoff. If the gut is sluggish, inflamed, or out of balance, the relay breaks down. Waste that was meant to leave can end up circling back into the bloodstream instead. The body finds itself processing the same compounds over and over, creating frustration rather than relief.

This is why you can eat well, take supplements, and follow a detox protocol, yet still feel heavy, bloated, or stuck. The liver may be doing its job just fine. The problem is often further downstream.

Bile: More Than Just Fat Digestion

One of the liver's main tools for moving waste out is bile. Most people know bile as the stuff that helps digest fats. When you eat a meal with butter, olive oil, or avocado, the gallbladder squeezes bile into the small intestine to help break down and absorb those fats. That part is true and important.

But bile does something else that often gets overlooked. It acts as a delivery truck for waste. Many of the compounds the liver processes, including used-up hormones, cholesterol, and fat-soluble toxins, get loaded into bile and sent to the intestines. The expectation is simple: these compounds will travel through the gut and leave the body in stool.

When everything moves at a healthy pace, this system works beautifully. Bile arrives, delivers its cargo, and the waste exits within a day or two. But when things slow down, the system runs into trouble.

When Waste Gets Recycled Instead of Removed

Here is a problem that does not get talked about enough: when stool sits in the colon too long, some of the waste it carries can be pulled back into the bloodstream.

The technical name for this is enterohepatic circulation, which simply means "gut-to-liver recycling." Certain compounds, especially hormones and their byproducts, can be reabsorbed through the intestinal wall if they hang around too long. Instead of leaving, they return to the liver, which then has to process them all over again[36].

This recycling effect helps explain something that puzzles many people: why they can feel burdened even when they think they are doing everything right. The liver might be working perfectly. But if the gut is not moving waste out efficiently, the liver's output just keeps coming back.

Hormone balance is especially sensitive to this. Estrogen, for example, is processed by the liver and sent out through bile. If gut transit is slow, estrogen metabolites can be reabsorbed instead of eliminated. This can contribute to symptoms of estrogen excess even when the body is not actually producing too much. The issue is not overproduction. It is under-elimination.

The takeaway is straightforward: detox cannot succeed if elimination is blocked. Opening exit routes matters as much as supporting the liver.

The Gut Is More Than a Tube

When most people picture the digestive system, they imagine a long tube that food travels through. That image is not wrong, but it misses something important. The gut is not just a passive pipeline. It is a living, active environment that plays a direct role in how well detox works.

Inside your intestines lives a community of trillions of bacteria, fungi, and other microorganisms. Together, they are called the gut microbiome. These tiny inhabitants are not just passengers. They influence digestion, immune function, mood, inflammation, and yes, detox.

Certain bacteria help regulate bile acids and support regular bowel movements. Others produce compounds that nourish the gut lining and keep it healthy. Some bacteria can even help bind and neutralize certain toxins, making them easier to eliminate. When the microbiome is balanced, it quietly supports detox in ways most people never notice[8].

But when the microbiome falls out of balance, things can shift in the wrong direction. Some bacterial patterns actually increase toxin recycling instead of reducing it. Others slow gut movement or raise inflammation. An imbalanced microbiome can make detox harder even when diet and lifestyle seem on point.

This is one reason why two people can follow the same detox approach and have completely different results. Their microbiomes are different. What supports one person's elimination may not be enough for another.

Bowel Movements Tell a Story

It is not the most glamorous topic, but bowel movements offer one of the clearest windows into how well detox is flowing.

Regular, comfortable elimination suggests that bile-bound waste is moving out as it should. The system is flowing. The relay is completing. When bowel movements are infrequent, difficult, or incomplete, it usually means waste is sitting longer than it should. The opportunity for recycling increases. Burden builds.

Research backs this up. Studies on gut transit time show that slower movement through the intestines gives more opportunity for compounds to be reabsorbed. People with longer transit times tend to have higher levels of certain recycled substances in their blood[28]. In simple terms: the longer waste sits, the more work the liver has to redo.

What does healthy elimination look like? Generally, one to three bowel movements per day, with stool that is well-formed but not hard, and easy to pass without straining. If you are going every two or three days, or if you regularly feel like you have not fully emptied, that is a sign the exit route needs attention.

Constipation: The Overlooked Bottleneck

Many people normalize constipation, especially when it develops slowly over time. They assume going every other day is just how their body works. But from a detox perspective, constipation is one of the most common and most underestimated problems.

When stool moves slowly, several things happen. First, water gets pulled out of it, making it harder and more difficult to pass. Second, the compounds in that stool, including the ones the liver carefully packaged for removal, have more time to be reabsorbed. Third, the gut environment can shift, with certain bacteria thriving in ways that do not support healthy elimination.

The result is a backup. Even if someone is eating clean, drinking water, and taking supplements, constipation can quietly undermine all of it. The front end of detox is working, but the back end is blocked.

This is why many people experience noticeable improvement simply by getting their bowels moving regularly. They did not need a fancier protocol or more supplements. They needed to open the exit.

The Gut Lining Matters Too

Beyond transit time and the microbiome, there is another factor that influences detox: the integrity of the gut lining itself.

The intestinal wall is designed to be selective. It lets nutrients through into the bloodstream while keeping unwanted substances contained within the digestive tract. Think of it like a smart filter that knows what to allow and what to block.

When this barrier gets damaged or "leaky," its selectivity decreases. Substances that should stay in the gut can slip through into the bloodstream. This triggers immune responses and raises inflammation throughout the body. Research consistently links increased gut permeability with inflammatory stress and broader health challenges[3].

From a detox standpoint, a leaky gut creates a double problem. More unwanted compounds enter circulation, increasing the load on the liver. At the same time, the inflammation that results makes it harder for detox systems to work efficiently. The body ends up fighting on two fronts.

What damages the gut lining? Chronic stress, alcohol, certain medications, processed foods, food sensitivities, and an imbalanced microbiome can all play a role. Healing the gut often involves removing irritants, supporting the microbiome, and giving the lining time and nutrients to repair.

Traditional Practices That Supported Elimination

Traditional food cultures did not have scientific terms for microbiome balance or gut permeability. But they practiced habits that supported elimination naturally, often without thinking of it as "detox" at all.

Many African dietary traditions emphasized whole plant foods, roots, and tubers. These foods are naturally rich in fiber, which plays several important roles in the gut. Fiber helps form stool, giving it the bulk it needs to move through the intestines. It also binds to bile and the waste it carries, helping ensure those compounds leave the body rather than getting recycled[41].

Fermented foods were common in many traditional diets as well. Fermentation was originally a preservation method, but it had side benefits for health. Fermented vegetables, grains, and beverages introduced beneficial bacteria into the gut, supporting the microbiome long before anyone knew the microbiome existed.

Meals were often simple and repetitive. This reduced the variety of compounds the gut had to process at any given time. When the digestive system sees the same familiar foods day after day, it can work more efficiently. Constant novelty, on the other hand, requires constant adaptation.

Movement was built into daily life. Walking, carrying, squatting, and working all helped stimulate gut movement. Physical activity encourages the muscular contractions that push stool through the intestines. Sedentary living, which is common today, removes this natural support.

These practices worked not because they were dramatic, but because they were steady. They supported elimination as a natural part of daily rhythm rather than something that required special intervention.

Supporting Elimination Without Force

The gut responds best to gentle, consistent support rather than aggressive intervention. Harsh laxatives and extreme fasting can irritate the digestive tract, disrupt the microbiome, and create dependency rather than true improvement. They might produce short-term movement, but they often make the underlying situation worse over time.

A more sustainable approach starts with the basics. Consistent hydration keeps stool soft and easier to pass. Fiber-rich whole foods give stool bulk and support the microbiome. Regular movement stimulates the gut's natural contractions. Simple meals reduce digestive burden. Reducing ultra-processed foods removes irritants and additives that can inflame the gut lining.

Stress management matters too. The gut and brain communicate constantly through what scientists call the gut-brain axis. When stress is high, digestive function often decreases. The body shifts resources away from digestion and toward dealing with the perceived threat. Chronic stress can slow gut transit, reduce beneficial bacteria, and increase inflammation. Calming the nervous system often helps the gut function better[30].

If constipation persists despite these foundations, it may be worth exploring further with a healthcare provider. Sometimes underlying issues like thyroid imbalance, pelvic floor dysfunction, or food sensitivities are contributing factors that need specific attention.

The Gut and Liver Work Together

The gut and liver are not separate players. They function as a tightly connected system. What happens in one directly affects the other.

When elimination improves, liver detox becomes easier. The liver can send waste out through bile, confident that it will actually leave. When the gut is inflamed or sluggish, waste gets recycled, and the liver's workload increases. It finds itself processing the same compounds again and again.

This connection explains why focusing only on the liver often produces limited results. You can take all the liver-supporting supplements in the world, but if elimination is blocked, the benefits will be modest at best. Detox works best when both systems are supported together.

Elimination is not something to fix once and forget. It reflects daily rhythm and long-term balance. The habits that support good elimination, like hydration, fiber, movement, and stress management, are the same habits that support overall health. They do not require obsession. They require consistency.

With elimination clearly understood, the next step is to explore another major factor that shapes detox capacity: metabolic stability. In the next chapter, we look at how blood sugar balance and inflammation influence the body's ability to detox smoothly and consistently.

When the exit is clear, everything flows better. That is the foundation elimination provides.

CHAPTER 5

Metabolic Stability, Blood Sugar, and Detox

Detox does not happen in a vacuum. It unfolds inside a living system that is constantly reading signals and deciding how to respond. Among the most powerful of those signals is blood sugar. When blood sugar is steady, detox pathways work quietly in the background. When blood sugar swings up and down throughout the day, detox becomes harder, slower, and more taxing, even when everything else seems to be in place.

This connection surprises many people. Blood sugar is usually discussed in the context of diabetes or weight management, not detox. But the body does not separate these systems the way textbooks do. Everything is connected. And blood sugar stability turns out to be one of the most overlooked foundations of effective detox.

Why Blood Sugar Matters for Detox

Every cell in your body needs energy to function. That energy comes primarily from glucose, a simple sugar that circulates in the blood. When glucose arrives at cells in a steady, predictable way, the body stays calm. Systems operate smoothly. Resources are available for maintenance tasks like repair, immune function, and detox.

When glucose levels spike and crash, the body interprets that pattern as instability. And instability triggers a stress response.

Think of it like driving a car. Smooth, consistent acceleration is easy on the engine. Constant speeding up and slamming on the brakes wears everything out faster. The body works the same way. It prefers steady energy delivery over dramatic swings.

Here is the key point: detox is not an emergency function. It is a maintenance function. The body always prioritizes immediate survival first. If blood sugar is crashing and stress hormones are spiking, the body focuses on stabilizing energy, not on long-term cleanup. Repair, elimination, and detox get pushed to the back of the line.

This means that someone with unstable blood sugar may struggle with detox even if they are eating clean foods and following a solid protocol. The instability itself is creating interference.

The Spike-and-Crash Cycle

To understand how blood sugar affects detox, it helps to see what happens during a typical spike-and-crash cycle.

Imagine eating a meal that is mostly refined carbohydrates: white bread, sweetened cereal, a pastry, or a sugary drink. These foods break down quickly into glucose, which floods into the bloodstream. Blood sugar rises rapidly.

In response, the pancreas releases insulin, a hormone that helps move glucose out of the blood and into cells. When blood sugar rises fast, insulin rises fast too. The goal is to bring things back to normal as quickly as possible.

But here is where problems start. A large insulin surge can overshoot. It pulls so much glucose out of the blood that levels drop too low. Now you are in a crash. Energy dips. The brain, which runs almost entirely on glucose, starts sending alarm signals. You feel tired, irritable, foggy, or suddenly hungry again, even though you just ate.

To rescue blood sugar from this low point, the body releases stress hormones like cortisol and adrenaline. These hormones tell the liver to release stored glucose, bringing levels back up. Crisis averted, at least temporarily.

But this rescue operation has costs. Stress hormones increase inflammation. They shift the body into a defensive mode that is not ideal for detox. And if this cycle repeats multiple times a day, day after day, the cumulative effect is significant.

Insulin Resistance and the Detox Connection

When blood sugar spikes happen repeatedly over months and years, something else begins to shift. Cells start becoming less responsive to insulin. They have been flooded with it so often that they begin to ignore the signal. This is called insulin resistance.

Insulin resistance is a spectrum, not an on-off switch. Someone can have mildly reduced insulin sensitivity without being diabetic. In fact, many people walk around with some degree of insulin resistance without knowing it. They just feel tired after meals, crave sugar, struggle with stubborn weight, or have energy that seems to drop in the afternoon.

From a detox perspective, insulin resistance creates several problems. First, it tends to increase inflammation. Research shows a strong link between reduced insulin sensitivity and higher levels of inflammatory markers in the body[5]. Second, it increases oxidative stress, which means more reactive molecules that the body must neutralize. Third, it keeps stress hormones elevated more often, which shifts resources away from maintenance functions like detox.

The result is a body that is constantly managing instability rather than efficiently clearing waste. Detox capacity gets crowded out.

Inflammation: The Resource Competition

Inflammation deserves special attention because it competes directly with detox for the same resources.

When the body is inflamed, whether from blood sugar swings, processed foods, stress, or other sources, it diverts energy, nutrients, and cellular attention toward managing that inflammation. Antioxidants get used up faster. Certain minerals and amino acids that the liver needs for detox get redirected. The immune system stays on higher alert, which consumes resources that might otherwise support repair and elimination.

Research confirms that chronic, low-grade inflammation is associated with impaired metabolic function and increased burden across multiple body systems 15. In this state, detox does not stop entirely, but it slows. Waste circulates longer. Symptoms can appear without a clear explanation.

The connection between blood sugar instability and inflammation creates a reinforcing cycle. Unstable blood sugar increases inflammation. Inflammation makes blood sugar harder to control. Each problem feeds the other. Breaking this cycle often requires addressing both sides at once.

Fat Tissue and Toxin Storage

Blood sugar instability also affects how the body handles stored toxins.

As discussed in earlier chapters, many environmental compounds are fat-soluble. The body stores them in fat tissue as a protective strategy, keeping them away from vital organs. Under stable conditions, these stored compounds release slowly and the liver can manage them without drama.

But when blood sugar is unstable, fat storage and fat breakdown become erratic too. Stress hormones like cortisol promote fat accumulation in certain areas while also triggering fat release at unpredictable times. This means stored toxins can be mobilized suddenly, flooding the system faster than the liver is prepared to handle.

This helps explain why some people feel worse when they start a detox program while also restricting calories dramatically. The combination of stress from caloric restriction plus unstable blood sugar can release stored compounds too quickly. The liver gets overwhelmed. Symptoms increase instead of decreasing.

Stabilizing blood sugar first creates a safer foundation for detox. When energy is steady and stress hormones are calm, fat tissue releases stored compounds at a pace the body can actually manage.

The Role of Meal Timing

Beyond what you eat, when you eat also sends powerful signals to the body.

Constant eating keeps insulin elevated throughout the day. The body stays in "processing mode" rather than shifting into repair and maintenance modes. Digestion runs continuously. The liver is always managing incoming fuel. There is little downtime for deeper cleanup work.

Structured eating patterns create different signals. When there are clear breaks between meals, insulin levels rise and fall as designed. During those lower-insulin windows, the body can shift attention toward repair, immune function, and detox. The liver gets time to catch up on processing rather than constantly dealing with new arrivals.

Research on time-restricted eating shows that even without changing what people eat, simply eating within a defined window (for example, 8 to 10 hours) can improve insulin sensitivity and reduce inflammatory markers 6. The body responds well to rhythm. It responds less well to chaos.

This does not mean everyone needs to fast aggressively or skip meals. For some people, especially those with blood sugar issues or high stress, skipping meals can backfire. The point is that eating should have a rhythm rather than being a continuous, all-day activity. Three meals with minimal snacking often works well. What matters most is consistency.

Traditional Patterns and Modern Disruption

Traditional food cultures understood rhythm intuitively, even without scientific language to explain it.

Meals were eaten at predictable times, often tied to the rhythms of work and rest. Snacking was limited not by discipline but by circumstance. Food was prepared fresh and eaten at defined meals rather than grabbed constantly throughout the day. The body knew what to expect and could prepare accordingly.

Foods themselves were different too. Whole grains, roots, legumes, and vegetables release their sugars slowly. They do not produce the sharp spikes that refined and processed foods create. Meals that included protein, fat, and fiber naturally slowed digestion and steadied blood sugar response. These were not calculated strategies. They were simply how food was prepared and eaten.

Modern eating patterns often disrupt this rhythm completely. Ultra-processed foods are designed to encourage frequent consumption. They combine refined carbohydrates, added sugars, and engineered flavors that override normal satiety signals. Snacking has become constant. Eating has become entertainment, stress relief, and background activity rather than a defined event.

The result is a body that never quite knows what to expect. Insulin stays elevated. Stress responses stay primed. Detox gets deprioritized because the system is always reacting to the latest input rather than settling into steady maintenance.

Stabilizing Blood Sugar Supports Everything

The good news is that blood sugar stability does not require extreme measures. It requires consistency.

Building meals around whole foods is the most important step. Protein, fiber, and healthy fats all slow digestion and prevent the rapid glucose spikes that refined foods create. A meal that includes some protein (eggs, fish, meat, legumes), some fiber (vegetables, whole grains), and some fat (olive oil, avocado, nuts) will produce a much steadier blood sugar response than a meal built mostly on refined carbohydrates.

Eating at regular times helps the body anticipate and prepare. The digestive system works better when it knows roughly when food is coming. Hormones involved in blood sugar regulation can calibrate more effectively when meals follow a predictable pattern.

Reducing or eliminating sugary drinks makes a significant difference. Liquid sugar hits the bloodstream faster than almost anything else. Sodas, sweetened teas, fruit juices, and specialty coffee drinks can spike blood sugar even when the rest of the diet seems reasonable.

Managing stress matters too. Stress hormones raise blood sugar independently of what you eat. Someone under chronic stress may struggle with blood sugar stability even on a clean diet. Addressing the stress itself, not just the food, becomes part of the solution.

Sleep plays a role as well. Poor sleep reduces insulin sensitivity and makes blood sugar harder to control the following day[42]. Prioritizing rest is not separate from metabolic health. It is foundational to it.

When blood sugar stabilizes, many things improve at once. Energy becomes steadier. Cravings soften. Mood becomes more predictable. Inflammation quiets. And detox stops being an uphill battle because the body finally has the stability it needs to do its maintenance work effectively.

With metabolic stability in place, the next step is to look more closely at how food itself communicates with the body. In the next chapter, we explore food as information and examine how daily dietary choices shape detox capacity in practical, sustainable ways.

CHAPTER 6

Food as Information, Not Just Fuel

For most of modern life, food has been reduced to numbers. Calories in, calories out. Grams of protein, fat, and carbohydrates. Eat less, move more. These ideas are not entirely wrong, but they are incomplete. They miss something important about how the body actually works.

Food is not just fuel. Food is information. Every meal sends messages that shape hormones, digestion, inflammation, and the body's ability to detox. When you eat, you are not just filling a tank. You are communicating with your biology.

This shift in perspective changes everything about how detox should be approached. The question is no longer just "How much should I eat?" It becomes "What signals am I sending?"

Beyond Calories

The calorie model treats the body like a simple machine. Put energy in, burn energy out, and the difference determines whether you gain or lose weight. There is some truth to this, but it tells only a small part of the story.

Consider two meals with the same number of calories. One is a plate of grilled salmon, roasted vegetables, and a small portion of rice. The other is a large soda and a bag of chips. Both might contain 500 calories, but the body responds to them completely differently.

The salmon meal delivers protein that the liver will use for detox processes. It provides fats that support hormone production and cell membranes. The vegetables offer fiber that feeds gut bacteria and binds waste for elimination. The whole meal digests slowly, producing a gentle rise in blood sugar and a calm, sustained energy release.

The soda and chips deliver a rapid sugar spike followed by a crash. They provide almost no fiber, protein, or micronutrients. They contain additives and industrial fats that the liver must process as foreign compounds. The body responds with inflammation, insulin surges, and stress signals. Same calories. Completely different messages. The body does not just count what comes in. It interprets what comes in and responds accordingly.

The Problem with Restriction

When food is treated only as fuel, detox often becomes an exercise in restriction. People cut calories, eliminate food groups, or jump from one set of rules to another, hoping that eating less will somehow lighten the burden. Sometimes this works in the short term. More often, it creates new problems.

The body interprets severe restriction as a signal of scarcity. When food becomes scarce, survival becomes the priority. The body slows metabolism, holds onto fat stores, and delays maintenance work like repair and detox. These are not malfunctions. They are intelligent responses to what the body perceives as a threat.

This is why aggressive dieting often backfires for detox. The very act of restriction can shift the body into a defensive state that makes elimination harder. Stress hormones rise. Digestion slows. The liver, deprived of nutrients it needs, cannot perform its binding and clearance work effectively.

When food is understood as information, the goal shifts. Instead of asking "How little can I eat?" you ask "What does my body need to hear?" The answer is usually not scarcity. It is nourishment, stability, and safety.

What the Liver Needs to Hear

The liver is one of the first organs to respond to dietary information. It sits at the crossroads of metabolism and detox, making constant decisions about how to use its resources.

When food arrives in a form the body recognizes, the liver works efficiently. Whole foods come with built-in context: fiber that slows absorption, minerals that support enzyme function, and compounds that guide digestion naturally. The liver knows what to do because the signals are clear.

When food arrives stripped of its natural structure and loaded with artificial additives, the liver faces a different challenge. Refined sugars hit the bloodstream too fast. Industrial fats require extra processing. Synthetic preservatives, colors, and flavor enhancers are foreign compounds that must be neutralized. The liver's workload increases while its support decreases.

This is not about moral judgment or food purity. It is about pattern recognition. The liver evolved processing foods that looked a certain way. When foods diverge too far from that pattern, more work is required to interpret and handle them.

Research consistently shows that dietary patterns built around whole foods are associated with lower inflammation and better metabolic function[22]. These outcomes are not accidents. They reflect the body responding to clear, recognizable signals rather than confusing ones.

Fiber: The Unsung Messenger

Fiber does not get the attention it deserves in most detox conversations. It is often treated as a "digestive" topic, something to think about if you are constipated but otherwise ignore. This misses how central fiber is to detox.

Fiber sends multiple messages at once. First, it slows the absorption of glucose, preventing the blood sugar spikes that disrupt metabolic stability. Second, it feeds beneficial bacteria in the gut, supporting a microbiome that aids detox. Third, it adds bulk to stool and binds to bile, helping ensure that waste actually leaves the body rather than being recycled.

When fiber is missing, all of these signals change. Blood sugar rises faster.

Gut bacteria shift toward less helpful populations. Stool moves more slowly, increasing the chance that compounds meant for elimination get reabsorbed instead.

Research confirms that adequate fiber intake supports bowel regularity, beneficial gut bacteria, and reduced recycling of waste compounds[41]. Traditional diets, built around whole plants, roots, and grains, naturally provided far more fiber than modern processed diets. This was not a calculated choice. It was simply how food was eaten.

Increasing fiber does not require complicated planning. Eating more vegetables, choosing whole grains over refined ones, including legumes, and snacking on fruit instead of processed foods will raise fiber intake naturally. The body responds quickly when this message changes.

Protein: Building Blocks for Detox

Protein is often discussed in terms of muscle building, but its role in detox is just as important.

The liver uses amino acids, the building blocks of protein, to perform its binding work in Phase II detoxification. Glycine, taurine, glutamine, and cysteine all play specific roles in neutralizing and packaging waste for elimination. Without adequate protein, the liver lacks raw materials, and detox slows regardless of what else you do.

Protein also sends satiety signals that help stabilize appetite and prevent the constant eating that keeps insulin elevated. A meal with adequate protein tends to satisfy longer than a meal built mostly on carbohydrates. This supports the meal spacing that gives the body time for repair and maintenance.

This does not mean you need to eat massive amounts of protein or follow a high-protein diet. It means protein should be present consistently at meals. Eggs at breakfast. Fish or chicken at lunch. Legumes or meat at dinner. The specific sources matter less than the consistency.

People who chronically under-eat protein often struggle with detox symptoms, fatigue, and slow recovery, even when their overall diet seems healthy. The body is missing a key message.

Fats: Messengers and Membranes

Dietary fats have been unfairly demonized for decades, and we are still recovering from the confusion this created. Fat is not the enemy. But the type and quality of fat matters enormously.

Fats serve as building materials for cell membranes, including the membranes of liver cells that perform detox. They are precursors to hormones that regulate inflammation, metabolism, and stress response. They help absorb fat-soluble vitamins that support detox pathways. And they stimulate bile release, which is essential for eliminating fat-soluble waste.

Traditional diets included fats in stable, minimally processed forms: animal fats, olive oil, coconut oil, fats from nuts and seeds. These fats supported the body without creating excessive oxidative stress. Modern diets are often dominated by industrial seed oils, extracted and refined using high heat and chemical solvents. These oils are high in omega-6 fatty acids and prone to oxidation. Research links excessive intake of these fats to increased inflammation and oxidative stress[40]. From a detox perspective, this creates more work for the body rather than supporting it.

The message here is not to fear fat, but to choose fats wisely. Olive oil, avocado, butter from grass-fed animals, coconut oil, and fats naturally present in whole foods support the body. Industrial oils found in fried foods, packaged snacks, and most restaurant cooking add burden.

Timing Sends Messages Too

When you eat communicates as much as what you eat.

Constant eating tells the body to stay in processing mode. Insulin remains elevated. Digestion never rests. The liver handles a continuous stream of incoming material and has little opportunity for deeper cleanup work.

Meals eaten at consistent times with clear breaks in between tell a different story. The body can anticipate when food is coming and prepare accordingly. Digestive enzymes and hormones calibrate to the rhythm. Between meals, insulin drops, and the body shifts into maintenance mode where repair and detox can happen more efficiently.

This does not require strict fasting or rigid rules. It requires rhythm. Three meals a day, eaten at roughly the same times, with minimal snacking in between, creates a pattern most bodies respond well to. The specifics can flex based on individual needs, but the underlying message of predictability and pauses is what matters.

Reducing Dietary Noise

Many modern detox struggles are not caused by a single toxin or a single bad food. They arise from constant dietary noise.

Ultra-processed foods combine refined carbohydrates, industrial fats, additives, and engineered flavors in ways the body struggles to interpret. Every meal becomes a puzzle. The liver is constantly adapting to unfamiliar combinations. The gut faces ingredients it does not recognize. Blood sugar swings. Inflammation rises. The signals are confusing rather than clear.

Traditional food cultures did the opposite. Meals were simple and repetitive. The same staple foods appeared day after day, prepared in familiar ways. This was not a lack of creativity. It was metabolic wisdom. When the body sees the same foods regularly, it processes them more efficiently. Digestion improves. Blood sugar response becomes more predictable. The system can relax.

Reducing dietary noise does not require perfection or rigid rules. It requires simplicity. Fewer ingredients. More whole foods. Less novelty. When meals are built from recognizable foods prepared simply, the body receives clear signals. Detox stops feeling like an uphill battle.

Food as Cooperation

At its core, detox is not about control. It is about cooperation. Food is one of the most powerful tools for building that cooperation.

When meals communicate safety and stability, the body shifts out of defensive mode. Energy becomes steadier. Cravings quiet down. Digestion improves. Elimination becomes more regular. Detox stops being something you have to force because the conditions that support it are already present.

This perspective takes pressure off. You do not have to find the perfect diet or eliminate every imperfect food. You have to send clearer signals more often than confusing ones. Over time, the body responds.

With this understanding in place, the next step is to move from principle to practice. In the next chapter, we explore how to structure detox-supportive meals that reduce burden while remaining simple, nourishing, and realistic for everyday life.

CHAPTER 7

Building Detox-Supportive Meals That Work

There is a moment that comes for almost everyone who starts learning about detox. You understand the concepts. You know about the liver and the gut and the importance of blood sugar stability. You have absorbed the science, and it all makes sense.

And then you stand in your kitchen at 6:30 in the evening and realize that knowledge alone does not make dinner.

This is where detox becomes real. Not in the theory, but in the repetition. Not in a perfect plan, but in the meals you can actually cook, eat, and return to day after day without effort or anxiety.

Detox-supportive eating is not about chasing the cleanest ingredients or designing meals that look impressive. It is about reducing friction. When friction is low, the body settles. When the body settles, detox becomes easier. The goal is not to micromanage nutrition. It is to create meals that quietly support the body's natural cleanup systems while still fitting into a normal life.

One Simple Intention

A detox-supportive meal begins with one simple intention: make the body's job easier, not harder.

That usually means moving away from meals that spike blood sugar, irritate digestion, or overload the liver with additives and processed fats. It means leaning toward meals that are balanced, predictable, and built from foods the body recognizes.

This does not require perfection. It does not require expensive ingredients or hours in the kitchen. It requires a framework that you can return to again and again, adjusting based on what is available and what sounds appealing.

When you have a framework, decisions become easier. You stop reinventing the wheel at every meal. You stop wondering whether you are doing it right. The structure carries you, and meals start supporting detox automatically.

The Detox Meal Triangle

If you want a simple mental model for building detox-supportive meals, think of a triangle with three points: protein, fiber, and fat.

Protein anchors the meal. It slows digestion. It steadies blood sugar response. It signals satisfaction so the body does not keep searching for more. And most importantly for detox, protein supplies amino acids that the liver uses to bind and neutralize waste.

Fiber guides elimination. It helps form stool, supports regular bowel movements, and binds compounds in the gut so they can leave the body rather than being recycled. Fiber also feeds beneficial gut bacteria, which play their own role in supporting detox.

Fat stabilizes. It slows the release of glucose into the bloodstream. It supports hormone production and helps absorb fat-soluble vitamins. It stimulates bile flow, which is one of the liver's main exit routes for waste. A meal with adequate fat tends to satisfy longer and produce steadier energy. When all three points of the triangle are present, the meal tends to land softly in the body. Blood sugar stays stable. Digestion proceeds calmly. Elimination moves along. When one point is missing, the body compensates, often with stress.

A meal of plain pasta with tomato sauce might taste fine, but it is mostly carbohydrate with little protein, fat, or fiber. Blood sugar spikes and crashes. Hunger returns quickly. Detox gets no support. Add grilled chicken, a side of sautéed vegetables, and a drizzle of olive oil, and the same pasta becomes a balanced meal. The triangle is complete.

Simplicity Over Complexity

Most people assume that detox eating must be complicated. They imagine elaborate recipes, rare ingredients, and hours of preparation. They build grocery lists that look like treasure hunts. They try to make every meal perfectly optimized.

What often happens is the opposite of what they intended. Complexity creates stress. Decision fatigue sets in. Consistency breaks. The body receives mixed signals because the approach cannot be sustained.

Traditional cultures often ate from a small rotation of staple meals. The same grains, the same vegetables, the same proteins appeared day after day, prepared in familiar ways. Repetition was not a lack of imagination. It was stability. When meals are familiar, the body becomes more efficient at processing them. Insulin response becomes more predictable. Digestion becomes more reliable. The nervous system relaxes because it recognizes the pattern.

This is why a few reliable meals beat a perfect plan you cannot sustain. Five or six meals that you can prepare without thinking, that you genuinely enjoy, and that check the boxes of the detox triangle will serve you better than an elaborate system that falls apart after two weeks.

Start simple. Build a small library of go-to breakfasts, lunches, and dinners. Rotate through them. Once that foundation is stable, you can add variety gradually if you want. But the foundation comes first.

Rhythm and Timing

Meal timing supports detox in ways that food composition alone cannot.

The body responds well to rhythm. When meals happen at roughly consistent times, digestive hormones, appetite signals, and elimination rhythms become more predictable. The body learns when to expect food and can prepare accordingly. Enzymes are ready. Blood flow shifts toward digestion. The process proceeds smoothly.

When eating is erratic, or when snacking becomes constant, the system stays switched on. Insulin remains elevated. Digestion never fully completes. The body spends more time managing incoming food and less time on repair and cleanup. Detox gets pushed to the background.

This does not mean you must eat at exact times every day or that flexibility is forbidden. It means meals work better as defined events rather than continuous grazing. Breakfast, lunch, and dinner with minimal snacking in between gives the body clear signals and natural pauses.

If you find yourself hungry between meals, that is often a sign that the previous meal was missing something. Usually protein or fat. Adjusting the meal itself tends to work better than adding snacks.

Portion Size: Satisfied, Not Stuffed

How much you eat matters, but not in the way diet culture usually presents it.

Overeating creates digestive burden. When too much food arrives at once, the stomach stretches, digestion slows, and the liver faces a larger processing load than it can handle efficiently. Energy that could go toward repair and cleanup gets diverted toward managing the excess. Bloating, fatigue, and sluggishness often follow.

Undereating creates different problems. It signals scarcity, which can increase stress hormones and cravings. It deprives the liver of nutrients it needs. It leaves you hungry between meals, which often leads to snacking on whatever is convenient.

Detox-supportive meals aim for the middle: satisfied, not stuffed. Nourished, not deprived. You should be able to finish a meal and feel content for several hours without thinking about food. If you feel uncomfortably full, the portion was probably too large. If you are hungry an hour later, something was missing.

Learning to recognize this middle ground takes time, especially if years of dieting or emotional eating have confused the signals. But the body knows how to regulate appetite when it receives consistent, balanced meals. Trust rebuilds gradually.

How You Cook Matters

The ingredients can be perfect, and the cooking method can still add burden.

When foods are cooked at very high temperatures, certain compounds form that increase oxidative stress and inflammation in the body. Scientists call these advanced glycation end products, or AGEs. They form especially during deep frying, heavy charring, and prolonged high-heat grilling. Research links high dietary AGE intake with increased inflammatory markers and metabolic stress[45].

This does not mean you can never grill or enjoy crispy food. It means your baseline cooking can lean toward gentler methods. Steaming, simmering, stewing, poaching, and roasting at moderate temperatures all preserve nutrients while producing fewer problematic compounds. These methods also tend to be simpler and require less active attention.

Marinating foods before high-heat cooking can reduce AGE formation. Using moisture, like braising meat or adding sauce, also helps. The goal is not perfection but awareness. If every meal involves deep frying or blackened edges, the cumulative effect matters. If gentler cooking is your default and high-heat methods are occasional, you are in a good place.

Fermented Foods: Gentle Support

Fermented foods can add support to a detox-focused diet, though they are not required for everyone.

Fermentation is an ancient preservation method that also changes food in beneficial ways. Bacteria and yeasts break down sugars and produce acids, enzymes, and other compounds that can support digestion and gut health.

Traditional cultures around the world developed their own fermented staples: kimchi, sauerkraut, miso, kefir, yogurt, fermented porridges, and countless others.

For detox, fermented foods offer a few potential benefits. They introduce beneficial bacteria that can support a healthy gut microbiome. They may improve digestion by providing enzymes and pre-digested nutrients. Some fermented foods are also good sources of fiber.

That said, fermented foods are not always comfortable for everyone, especially at first. If you are not used to them, introducing large amounts suddenly can cause gas, bloating, or digestive upset. The key is gentle introduction. A small amount consistently is often better than a large amount that causes discomfort.

If fermented foods feel good and you enjoy them, include them regularly. If they do not agree with you, do not force it. They are a support, not a requirement.

The State You Eat In

There is another layer to meals that most detox conversations ignore: the state you are in while eating.

Digestion is not only chemistry. It is also nervous system. When you eat in a rush, while anxious, while scrolling your phone, while working, or while standing at the counter, the body reads that state as stress. Stress shifts the body away from "rest and digest" mode and toward a defensive posture. In this stressed state, blood flow moves away from the digestive organs. Enzyme production decreases. Gut movement slows. The same meal can land very differently depending on whether you eat it calmly or consume it under pressure[7].

This is why detox-supportive meals are not only about the plate. They are about the pace. Sitting down. Taking a breath before the first bite. Eating without urgency. Chewing thoroughly. Letting your body recognize that food is arriving and that there is no threat.

This shift does not require elaborate rituals or perfect stillness. It requires a few moments of transition. Put the phone away. Sit at a table if possible. Notice the food in front of you. These small changes signal safety to the nervous system and allow digestion to proceed as it should.

Building Your Meal Library

If detox-supportive eating feels like a constant mental project, it will not last. The most effective approach is one that requires minimal daily decisions.

Start by identifying a few reliable options for each meal. Two or three breakfasts you genuinely enjoy that include protein, fiber, and fat. Three or four lunches that are easy to prepare or bring with you. Four or five dinners that you can rotate through without getting bored.

These do not need to be fancy. Eggs with vegetables and toast. A salad with grilled chicken and olive oil. Baked fish with roasted vegetables. Soup with beans and greens. Simple combinations that check the boxes.

Once you have this library, meal planning becomes rotation rather than invention. You know what works. You keep the ingredients on hand. Decisions disappear. Consistency becomes automatic.

From this stable foundation, variety can be added gradually if you want. New recipes can be tested on weekends or when energy allows. But the foundation carries you during busy weeks, stressful seasons, and times when willpower is low.

This approach aligns naturally with the principles in the 15-Day Detox Planner. The planner emphasized hydration, whole foods, regular meals, movement, and reflection. Those habits reduce strain without requiring obsession. They create rhythm. And when rhythm returns, the body often responds in quiet, satisfying ways.

Meals do not need to be labeled as "detox meals" to support detox. They only need to reduce friction. When friction is low, the body does the rest. With meal foundations in place, the next step is to explore additional supports that can strengthen this process without overwhelming it. In the next chapter, we turn to herbs, roots, and targeted supplements: not as shortcuts, but as gentle tools that work best when the food foundation is already strong.

CHAPTER 8

Herbs, Roots, and Targeted Support

There is a certain point in every detox journey when the foundation starts to feel steady. Meals become simpler. Digestion becomes more predictable. Elimination improves. The mind quiets down because the body no longer feels like a constant project.

And then curiosity shows up.

If food and rhythm can create this much change, what happens when you add herbs, roots, and targeted support? What happens when you bring in the plant wisdom that traditional systems have used for generations?

This is a natural curiosity, and it deserves a thoughtful answer. Used wisely, these tools can deepen the work that is already happening. Used carelessly, they can create the very stress that detox is trying to reduce.

Amplifiers, Not Shortcuts

A healthy approach to herbs and supplements begins with a simple truth: they are not shortcuts. They are amplifiers. They tend to make whatever is happening in the body more noticeable.

If your foundation is chaotic, with irregular meals, poor sleep, constipation, or high stress, adding strong herbal support can amplify the chaos. You might experience headaches, digestive upset, skin reactions, or fatigue. These are not signs that the herbs are "working." They are signs that the body is struggling to integrate something new while already under strain.

If your foundation is stable, with regular meals, good sleep, steady elimination, and manageable stress, gentle herbal support often feels like a smooth upgrade. Energy improves. Digestion gets a little easier. The body responds well because it has capacity to spare.

This is why the earlier chapters focused so heavily on food, blood sugar, elimination, and rhythm. Those are the foundations. Herbs and supplements are tools that work best when built on a solid base.

Traditional Wisdom About Plants

Traditional African healing systems understood plants differently than modern supplement culture does. Plants were not treated like isolated chemicals to be extracted and concentrated. They were treated like partners with their own intelligence and timing.

Dosage mattered. Seasons mattered. Timing mattered. The state of the person mattered. Healers did not typically stack ten plants at once hoping something would work. The focus was on balance, not intensity. On reading the body's responses and adjusting accordingly.

Bitter plants, for example, were often consumed before or with meals rather than in massive therapeutic doses. The bitterness itself was part of daily eating, woven into the rhythm of life rather than reserved for special interventions. This gentle, consistent approach supported digestion and elimination without creating drama.

Modern research helps explain why this approach works. Many traditional herbs influence detox indirectly, through digestion, bile flow, antioxidant activity, and inflammatory balance. They do not force toxins out. They support the conditions that allow the body to clear more efficiently on its own.

The Power of Bitterness

Bitterness is one of the clearest examples of how plants communicate with the body.

We often treat taste as simple preference, liking or disliking certain flavors. But taste is also information. The tongue is covered with receptors that detect different taste qualities, and bitterness triggers a specific set of responses.

What surprised modern scientists is that bitter taste receptors exist not only in the mouth but throughout the digestive tract. When bitter compounds reach these receptors, they trigger signals that influence gut hormones, gastric activity, and bile flow[10]. The body interprets bitterness as a cue to prepare for digestion.

This matters for detox because bile is not just for fat digestion. Bile is one of the liver's main exit routes for waste. When bile flows well, fat-soluble toxins and spent hormones move out through the gut more efficiently. Supporting healthy bile movement can reduce the recycling of waste compounds and support smoother elimination.

This is why bitter roots and leaves have held such an important place in traditional wellness systems. Dandelion root is a familiar example in modern herbal use. It contains bitter compounds that have been traditionally associated with digestive support and bile flow[12]. Burdock root is another example, long used for digestive and skin health, which makes sense when you remember that skin often reflects the state of internal elimination.

The key principle is that bitter plants work through signaling, not forcing. They wake the system up and encourage it to do what it already knows how to do. This is gentle support, not aggressive intervention.

Antioxidant and Anti-Inflammatory Support

A second category of herbal support involves antioxidant and anti-inflammatory plants.

Detox processes naturally involve chemical transformation. As the liver converts compounds from one form to another, reactive byproducts can be generated. These reactive molecules need to be neutralized, or they can cause cellular stress. The body has built-in antioxidant systems to handle this, but those systems can become depleted when burden is high or nutrient intake is low.

Plants rich in polyphenols and other antioxidant compounds can support this internal balancing act. They provide raw materials that help the body neutralize reactive molecules and manage inflammation.

Moringa is one example that has received significant research attention. It carries a dense nutritional profile along with compounds that have been studied for antioxidant and anti-inflammatory effects[34]. The key is not that moringa is a miracle. The key is that plants like moringa can support the calm, nourished internal environment that detox needs.

This category also includes teas that many people already enjoy. Hibiscus, rooibos, and green tea all contain compounds that support antioxidant activity. They are not dramatic interventions. They are daily supports that lower oxidative stress and provide steady plant compounds without overwhelming the system.

The goal with these plants is not to force change but to create conditions where detox can proceed with less friction.

Supporting Kidney Function

While the liver prepares waste and the gut eliminates a large portion through bile, the kidneys handle water-soluble waste. They filter the blood constantly, removing excess minerals, metabolic byproducts, and other compounds that dissolve in water.

Hydration is the most important support for kidney function. Without adequate water, the kidneys cannot filter efficiently. But certain plants have traditionally been used to support urinary flow and mineral balance as well.

Nettle leaf is commonly mentioned in this context, along with parsley and other mineral-rich greens. These plants have a long history of use for supporting fluid balance. Many African traditions include similar plants, often consumed as teas or incorporated into meals.

The key, again, is gentleness. The goal is not to force fluid out through harsh diuretics, which can deplete minerals and stress the kidneys. The goal is steady movement and steady replenishment. Drinking adequate water while including gentle supportive plants creates flow without strain.

Adaptogens and Stress

There is one category of herbal support that confuses people more than any other: adaptogens.

Adaptogens are often marketed like performance enhancers, promising more energy, sharper focus, and better endurance. But their traditional use is closer to resilience support. They help the body adapt to stress rather than eliminating stress entirely.

This matters for detox because stress is one of the most underappreciated detox disruptors. When stress is chronic, digestion slows, inflammation rises, elimination becomes sluggish, and hormone balance shifts. The body stays in a defensive posture that is not ideal for repair and cleanup. If the nervous system never settles, detox will always feel harder than it needs to.

Ashwagandha is one of the most studied adaptogens. Research reviews have found evidence that it can support stress regulation and reduce cortisol levels in some people[2]. Other adaptogens from various traditions offer similar potential, though individual responses vary.

This does not mean adaptogens are for everyone or that they should be taken indefinitely. It means stress regulation matters for detox, and certain plants may support that regulation when used appropriately. If the nervous system is stuck in overdrive, calming it down can make every other aspect of detox work better.

Supplements: Power and Restraint

Targeted supplements occupy a different space than whole herbs. They are concentrated, isolated, and powerful. This makes them potentially useful but also potentially problematic.

Whole plants come with natural buffers, with hundreds of compounds working together in ways we do not fully understand. When a single compound is extracted and concentrated, those buffers are often lost. The effect becomes more direct, but also more one-dimensional.

Nutrients like magnesium, zinc, B vitamins, and amino acids do play roles in detox pathways. The liver needs these building blocks to perform its binding and transformation work. For someone with genuine deficiency, targeted supplementation can make a real difference.

But the most common mistake people make with supplements is assuming that more is better. They stack multiple products hoping to cover all bases. When the body reacts with bloating, headaches, sleep disruption, or other symptoms, it becomes impossible to know what caused what.

The wiser approach is restraint. Add one thing at a time. Start with a low dose. Observe. If it helps, continue. If it creates problems, stop. Let the body guide decisions rather than following a checklist.

Timing and Cycling

When you take herbs and supplements matters almost as much as what you take.

Some supports work best with meals because digestion is active and bile is flowing. Bitter herbs taken before eating can prime the digestive system for what is coming. Fat-soluble nutrients absorb better when taken with food that contains fat.

Other supports work better between meals or at specific times of day. Adaptogens that affect energy might be better in the morning. Calming herbs might be better in the evening. Paying attention to timing often makes the difference between a supportive experience and an irritating one.

Cycling matters too. Traditional systems rarely used the same plant at the same dose indefinitely. Herbs were used for seasons, for specific phases, or in response to particular needs. Then they were set aside. This cycling allows the body to respond without becoming dependent or desensitized.

Modern supplement culture often ignores this wisdom, encouraging daily use of the same products month after month. The body may eventually stop responding, or imbalances may develop that were not present at the start. Building in breaks, whether a few days each week or a few weeks each season, respects how the body actually works.

The Simple Rule

If there is one rule to remember about herbal and supplement support, it is this: if adding something increases chaos, something is wrong.

The dose may be too high. The timing may be off. The foundation may not be as steady as it needs to be. Or that particular support may simply not be right for your body at this time.

Detox should become steadier over time, not more dramatic. If herbs and supplements are making things feel worse, that is not a sign to push harder. It is a sign to step back, reassess, and simplify.

Herbs and roots are not meant to replace meals or override poor foundations. They are meant to complement what is already working. A bitter tea before a meal, a mineral-rich herb in the evening, a gentle adaptogen during a stressful season: these are supports that work best when the basics are already in place.

When used with respect, these tools deepen the work that food and rhythm have started. They do not create detox. They make detox easier.

With that understanding in place, the next pathway becomes clear. If elimination is the exit route, circulation is the delivery system. In the next chapter, we turn our attention to movement, sweat, and lymphatic flow, and explore why the body clears waste through motion rather than stillness.

CHAPTER 9

Movement, Circulation, and Sweat

Detox is often imagined as something that happens while the body is still. A drink is consumed, a supplement is taken, a food is avoided, and then the body is expected to clean itself out somewhere in the background. But the human body was not built to detox in stillness alone. Detox is not only chemistry. It is flow. And flow depends on motion.

For most of human history, movement was not a separate activity. It was life. Walking to gather water, carrying supplies, tending fields, bending, squatting, reaching, and rising again. Movement was not punishment or performance. It was daily rhythm. And that rhythm quietly supported circulation, elimination, and balance in ways modern life often forgets.

Why Movement Matters for Detox

When people feel stuck during detox, heavy, puffy, sluggish, or foggy, it is tempting to assume the liver is struggling or the gut is blocked. Sometimes those are factors. But often the issue is simpler: the transport system is not moving.

The body has two main fluid transport systems. Blood circulation is the more familiar one. The heart pumps blood through arteries to deliver oxygen and nutrients, then pulls it back through veins to collect waste and return for another cycle. This system runs constantly and has its own powerful pump.

But there is a second system that most people know little about: the lymphatic system. This network of vessels runs alongside the blood vessels, collecting fluid, cellular debris, and waste products from tissues and moving them toward processing stations called lymph nodes. The lymphatic system plays a crucial role in immune function and in clearing certain types of waste from the body.

Here is the key difference: the lymphatic system does not have its own pump. Unlike the heart, which pushes blood whether you are moving or not, the lymphatic system depends entirely on external forces to move fluid. Those forces come from skeletal muscle contraction, breathing, and changes in pressure within the body[9].

In other words, when you move, lymph moves. When you stay still, lymph can stagnate.

This helps explain why gentle movement can create a kind of detox relief that food and supplements alone sometimes cannot. It is not magic. It is drainage.

The Muscle Pump

When muscles contract and relax, they squeeze the lymphatic vessels running through and around them. These vessels have one-way valves that prevent backflow, so each squeeze pushes fluid forward toward central collection points. Repeated muscle contractions create a pumping action that moves lymph steadily through the system.

This is why walking is one of the most effective detox supports available. The muscles of the legs contract rhythmically with each step, squeezing lymphatic vessels and pushing fluid upward. The movement also increases blood flow, which helps deliver oxygen to tissues and carry waste toward elimination organs.

Walking does not need to be intense to be effective. A moderate pace that you can sustain for twenty or thirty minutes produces steady pumping action without the stress that high-intensity exercise can create. After meals, a short walk can support digestion by increasing blood flow to the gut and encouraging gentle movement through the intestines.

This is also why prolonged sitting creates problems beyond just muscle stiffness. When you sit for hours without moving, the muscle pump essentially stops. Fluid accumulates in the lower legs. Lymph stagnates. The transport system that should be moving waste toward elimination is barely functioning.

Simply standing up and walking around for a few minutes every hour can make a meaningful difference. The body does not need marathon training. It needs regular activation.

Breathing as a Pump

Breathing plays a role in lymphatic flow that most people never consider.

The diaphragm is a dome-shaped muscle that sits below the lungs and above the abdominal organs. When you inhale, the diaphragm contracts and moves downward, creating negative pressure in the chest that draws air into the lungs. When you exhale, it relaxes and moves upward.

This up-and-down movement does more than move air. It creates pressure changes that affect fluid movement throughout the torso. The main lymphatic channel, called the thoracic duct, runs through the chest and empties into the bloodstream near the heart. Deep diaphragmatic breathing helps draw lymph upward through this channel and into circulation[37].

Most people breathe shallowly, using only the upper chest. Stress tightens the muscles around the ribs. Sitting collapses the posture. Over time, breathing becomes small, and the pumping action of the diaphragm diminishes.

Deep, slow breathing that engages the belly restores this pump. You can feel the difference: when you breathe deeply, the belly expands on the inhale and contracts on the exhale. This full movement massages the organs, stimulates the diaphragm, and supports lymph flow.

This makes deep breathing more than a relaxation technique. It is a physical support for drainage and circulation. A few minutes of intentional deep breathing can be surprisingly effective, especially when combined with gentle movement.

Strength and Metabolic Health

Strength-building movement matters for detox, though not for the reasons many people assume.

Muscle is one of the body's most important metabolic tissues. When muscles are active and well-maintained, they improve how the body handles glucose and responds to insulin. Strong muscles pull glucose out of the blood more efficiently, which helps stabilize blood sugar and reduces the metabolic stress that interferes with detox.

This does not mean you need to become a bodybuilder or spend hours in a gym. Functional movements that challenge muscles, like carrying groceries, climbing stairs, squatting to pick things up, or doing simple bodyweight exercises, provide the stimulus needed to maintain metabolic health.

Resistance training also supports bone health, posture, and the ability to stay active as you age. These benefits compound over time. The goal is not dramatic transformation but steady maintenance of the body's functional capacity.

Flexibility and Flow

Stretching and mobility work contribute to detox in their own way.

When tissues are tight, they restrict movement, compress vessels, and reduce the ease of circulation. A chronically tight hip flexor, for example, can compress lymphatic vessels in the groin area and impede drainage from the legs. Tight shoulders can restrict blood flow and lymphatic movement in the arms and upper body.

When tissues become more mobile and hydrated through regular stretching, flow improves. This is not just about flexibility in the traditional sense. It is about creating space for fluid to move and for the body to function without unnecessary restriction.

Posture fits into the same picture. Collapsed posture compresses the chest and abdomen, limiting both breathing depth and fluid movement through the torso. An upright posture with an open rib cage and relaxed shoulders reduces these barriers. The diaphragm can move more fully. The lungs can expand more completely. Circulation has fewer obstacles.

Simple daily stretching, even just five or ten minutes, can make a meaningful difference in how freely fluid moves through the body.

Sweat: A Supporting Exit Route

Sweat is often promoted as a major detox pathway, but the reality is more modest. The liver and kidneys handle the vast majority of waste elimination. Sweat is a supporting player, not the star.

That said, sweat does appear to excrete certain compounds that are difficult to eliminate through other routes. A systematic review of research on toxic metals in sweat found evidence that arsenic, cadmium, lead, and mercury can be excreted through sweat, though the amounts vary widely depending on exposure levels and sweating conditions[39].

This suggests that regular sweating can be a useful addition to a detox-supportive lifestyle, especially for people with higher toxic metal exposure. But it should not be treated as a replacement for liver and gut elimination, which remain the primary pathways.

What matters most is how sweating is approached. Many people swing between two extremes: no sweating at all, or intense sessions used as punishment. Detox responds best to moderation. A light sweat achieved regularly through movement or gentle heat often supports circulation and lymph flow more effectively than rare, extreme efforts.

Some people do well with sauna sessions. Others prefer brisk walks, cycling, or other movement that produces mild perspiration. Research comparing different sweating methods suggests that active sweating through exercise may support excretion somewhat differently than passive sweating through heat alone[25]. Both have value. The key is consistency rather than intensity.

Hydration becomes especially important when sweating regularly. Sweat carries water and minerals out of the body. Replacing both with adequate fluids and mineral-rich foods supports the body's ability to sweat without depleting itself.

The Emotional Side of Movement

There is also an emotional dimension to movement that affects detox.

Many people carry stress in the body as tension and stagnation. The shoulders hunch. The jaw clenches. The belly tightens. Over time, this chronic tension affects circulation, breathing, and the overall ease with which the body moves fluid.

Movement helps discharge this stored tension. A walk in nature can shift mood and relax the nervous system. Stretching can release physical holding patterns. Even shaking, dancing, or other spontaneous movement can help the body let go of accumulated stress.

This matters because chronic stress is one of the most consistent detox disruptors. When the nervous system stays in a defensive state, digestion slows, inflammation rises, and detox becomes harder. Movement that helps shift the nervous system from stress mode to calm mode supports detox indirectly by creating better internal conditions.

Detox-supportive movement is not about compensation or punishment. It is not about undoing a meal or earning the right to eat. It is about sending a daily signal that says: the system is awake, the pathways are open, and flow is allowed.

Making Movement Sustainable

The most effective approach to movement is integration rather than addition. Instead of trying to add a separate "exercise session" to an already full day, look for ways to weave movement into what you are already doing.

Short walks after meals support digestion and circulation. Standing breaks during work prevent the stagnation of prolonged sitting. Light stretching in the morning prepares the body for the day. A few minutes of deep breathing before bed helps transition into rest.

These small choices create a steady current in the body. They do not require gym memberships, special equipment, or large blocks of time. They require awareness and a willingness to move throughout the day rather than being sedentary for long stretches.

Over time, this steady current changes how detox feels. Elimination becomes easier. Puffiness and swelling reduce. Energy improves. The body feels less congested and more responsive. Detox stops feeling like something you have to push because the system is already moving.

With circulation and movement addressed, the final piece of the puzzle comes into view. Detox is not meant to be a one-time event. It is meant to become a way of living: steady, rhythmic, and sustainable. In the final chapter, we bring everything together and turn this blueprint into a long-term lifestyle that supports health without constant effort.

CHAPTER 10

Living the Blueprint

Detox is often treated as an event. A window of time. A challenge to complete and then move on from. But the deeper truth revealed throughout this book is simpler and far more sustainable: detox is not something you do once. It is something the body is always doing. The only real question is whether your daily life supports that work or quietly works against it.

By this point, detox should feel less mysterious and less dramatic. You have seen the body as a system: how the liver transforms, how the gut eliminates, how the kidneys filter, how the lymph moves, and how food and rhythm shape the environment those systems live in. None of these elements are extreme on their own. Together, they form a pattern.

That pattern is the blueprint.

From Phase to Pattern

There is a moment when the mindset shifts. It does not happen overnight, and it usually comes quietly. You stop thinking of health as a destination you reach through effort and start seeing it as something you maintain through simple, repeated choices. The difference feels subtle at first, but it changes everything.

When detox is treated as a phase, there is always a finish line somewhere ahead. You push through discomfort. You restrict. You count days until it is over. And when it ends, the relief feels like permission to return to old patterns. This is why so many people find themselves repeating the same cleanse or program every few months, stuck in a cycle of effort and collapse.

When detox is treated as a pattern, the finish line disappears. There is no dramatic end because there was no dramatic beginning. There are only habits that support the body and habits that work against it. The goal becomes steadiness, not intensity. Recovery becomes built-in rather than hoped for.

This shift requires letting go of the idea that more effort produces better results. In biology, effort often creates stress, and stress is something detox systems have to manage alongside everything else. A body pushed too hard has less energy left over for repair.

A blueprint is not a rigid plan. It is a guiding structure. It shows how pieces fit together so that decisions become easier, not harder. When detox becomes a lifestyle rather than a phase, it stops demanding constant attention. The body knows what to do because the environment around it is no longer confusing.

Why Stability Beats Speed

One of the most important shifts is moving away from the idea of "getting toxins out" as quickly as possible. Speed is rarely the goal in biological systems. Stability is.

Think of how the body handles other processes. Digestion takes hours because food needs to be broken down carefully, not rushed. Sleep happens in cycles because each stage serves a different purpose. Growth and repair follow rhythms that cannot be hurried without consequences. The body operates on its own timeline, and trying to force faster results usually backfires.

Detox follows the same principle. The liver processes compounds at a certain rate. Bile flows according to digestive signals. The kidneys filter blood constantly but cannot be sped up by willpower. The lymph moves only when the body moves. Each system has built-in limits that reflect careful biological engineering, not design flaws to be overridden.

When blood sugar is stable, digestion is supported, elimination is regular, and stress is managed, detox happens quietly in the background. When those foundations are unstable, no amount of intervention creates lasting change. The body returns to its baseline as soon as the intervention stops, because nothing fundamental has shifted.

This is why earlier chapters emphasized rhythm over restriction. Regular meals, consistent hydration, predictable movement, and reliable sleep cues signal safety. Safety allows the body to shift energy away from defense and toward repair. Repair is where detox thrives.

The Language of Awareness

A detox lifestyle does not require perfection. It requires awareness.

Awareness sounds abstract, but it shows up in small, practical ways. You notice when meals become rushed and digestion suffers. You notice when sitting all day leaves you feeling heavy and stagnant. You notice when stress tightens your breath and disrupts sleep. These observations are not failures. They are feedback.

The body is always communicating. Energy levels, mood, digestion, skin, sleep quality, mental clarity: these are all messages about how internal systems are handling their current load. When you learn to read these signals, you gain information that no test or scan can provide. You know, from the inside, whether things are moving in the right direction.

This kind of awareness takes practice. Most people have learned to ignore body signals in favor of schedules, obligations, and external expectations. Reconnecting with internal feedback is not about becoming obsessive or anxious. It is about restoring a basic form of self-knowledge that should never have been lost.

Simple questions build this awareness. How did I feel after that meal? How was my energy in the afternoon? How easily did I fall asleep? Did I wake up rested? These are not complicated questions, but answering them honestly creates a feedback loop that guides choices over time.

Instead of jumping into another cleanse, you return to the blueprint. You restore meal balance. You reintroduce gentle movement. You simplify food choices. You create space for rest. Detox resumes naturally because the conditions that support it are present again.

Programs Versus Lifestyles

This is the difference between a detox program and a detox lifestyle. Programs rely on compliance. Lifestyles rely on alignment.

Compliance means following rules created by someone else. It means willpower, discipline, and the constant feeling that you might be doing something wrong. Compliance works for short periods, but it creates tension. The moment pressure lets up, old habits return because nothing internal has changed.

Alignment means your habits work with the body's design rather than against it. There is no rule book to follow because the principles make sense. You eat in ways that support blood sugar because you understand what happens when blood sugar crashes. You move because you feel the difference when you do not. You rest because you recognize the cost of ignoring sleep.

Human physiology responds best to consistency, not constant novelty. The body prefers familiar foods prepared simply. It prefers daily movement rather than occasional intensity. It prefers regular sleep-wake cycles rather than constant disruption. These are not modern trends. They are built-in design features.

Alignment also creates flexibility. When life disrupts your routine, as it will, you are not knocked off course because you understand what matters most. You know which basics to return to. Recovery is not about starting over. It is about finding your way back to familiar ground.

Ancestral Rhythm Meets Modern Biology

From a traditional perspective, this is where ancestral wisdom quietly meets modern biology. Long before metabolic pathways were named, cultures organized life around cycles. Day and night, work and rest, feast and simplicity. These cycles supported balance without calling it "detox." Waste moved because life itself moved in rhythm.

Traditional African cultures knew this intuitively. Meals followed the sun. Activity followed necessity. Rest followed labor. Food was seasonal because it had to be, and the body adapted to those rhythms over generations. There were no detox products or special programs because the lifestyle itself was the program.

Modern research helps explain what tradition observed. Chronic inflammation is linked with broad metabolic dysfunction across the lifespan and can interfere with normal physiological balance[15]. Irregular eating patterns and constant blood sugar swings add stress that the body must manage on top of everything else[4]. Structured meal timing patterns such as time-restricted eating have been shown to improve metabolic markers, pointing to the importance of rhythm rather than intensity[43].

Sedentary living reduces lymphatic movement, since lymph flow depends heavily on body movement and pressure changes rather than a central pump[16]. Sleep disruption interferes with the brain's glymphatic system, which clears metabolic waste during rest[46]. Each of these findings confirms what traditional patterns already showed: rhythm matters.

The goal is not to recreate ancient life in a modern world. That would be impossible and, in many ways, undesirable. The goal is to extract the principles that made those rhythms effective and apply them in ways that fit current circumstances. Regular meals, daily movement, protected sleep, and occasional breaks from constant input. These adaptations honor the body's design without demanding a time machine.

Integration Across Life's Seasons

None of this is meant to create anxiety. It is meant to create clarity. What is often missing is integration.

Integration is what turns information into practice. It is the bridge between knowing and doing.

The blueprint integrates food, movement, herbs, and mindset into a single framework that can flex with real life. There will be seasons when support needs to be stronger: after illness, during high stress, or when exposure increases. There will be seasons when the foundation alone is enough. The goal is not to stay in detox mode forever. The goal is to know when support is needed and how to provide it gently.

Stress is a good example. During periods of high demand, the body shifts resources toward managing that stress. Digestion may slow. Sleep may suffer. Inflammation may rise. These are normal adaptive responses, not failures. But they also mean that detox capacity is temporarily reduced. Recognizing this allows you to respond appropriately: simplify food, prioritize rest, support elimination gently, and wait for the storm to pass.

Travel creates similar challenges. Time zone changes disrupt circadian rhythms. Unfamiliar food creates digestive uncertainty. Sitting for hours on planes or in cars slows lymphatic movement. A traveler who understands the blueprint does not panic. They stay hydrated, move when possible, eat simply, and give the body time to readjust.

Illness requires another adjustment. When the immune system is active, the body is already working hard. Adding aggressive detox protocols on top of that can overwhelm systems that need their energy elsewhere. The wiser approach is to support rest, provide nourishment, and let the body focus on recovery. Detox can resume when health returns.

This flexibility is the mark of a lifestyle rather than a program. You are not following a fixed script. You are responding to current conditions with a set of principles that adapt to circumstances.

Restraint as Wisdom

This is also where restraint becomes a form of wisdom. Knowing when not to add more is just as important as knowing what to add.

Modern wellness culture tends toward accumulation. More supplements, more protocols, more interventions. Each new product promises an edge, an improvement, a missing piece. The result is often a complicated routine that creates more stress than it solves, along with a nagging suspicion that you are still missing something.

Traditional wisdom moved in the opposite direction. Interventions were used when needed and removed when they were not. Plants were taken for seasons, not permanently. Intensity was reserved for specific situations, not daily life. The body was trusted to do its job when conditions were right.

When the body is responding well, with energy steady, digestion regular, sleep improving, intervention can often be reduced. The system is doing its job. This is success, even though it feels quiet. The absence of struggle is the goal, not a sign that you need to try harder.

Adding support makes sense when there are clear signals that the body needs help. Returning symptoms, persistent fatigue, digestive disruption, poor recovery from stress: these are invitations to revisit the blueprint and see what might be missing. But adding support just because it exists, or because someone recommended it, often creates confusion without benefit.

Measuring Success Differently

A detox lifestyle changes how success is measured. Instead of chasing rapid weight loss, dramatic symptoms, or short-term intensity, success becomes quieter. You measure it in resilience. In how quickly the body recovers after stress. In how easily you return to balance.

Resilience is not about never being affected by challenges. It is about how well you bounce back. A resilient body can handle a late night and recover its energy the next day. It can manage a rich meal without days of digestive upset. It can navigate stress without falling apart. These capacities are more meaningful than any cleanse result because they reflect true adaptability.

Adaptability is the long-term goal of the blueprint. Not a body that requires perfect conditions to function, but a body that can handle variation because its systems are fundamentally sound. This kind of health is not fragile. It does not require constant vigilance. It simply continues working because the foundation supports it.

The markers that matter most are often invisible. Steady energy through the day. Clear thinking. Predictable digestion. Solid sleep. Emotional steadiness. Consistent recovery from exertion. These are the signs that detox pathways are working, that inflammation is managed, that the body is operating within its design parameters.

When these markers are present, you do not need to think about detox very often. The system runs in the background, quietly clearing waste and maintaining balance while you live your life. That is the ultimate goal: health that requires less effort because it has been built on a solid foundation.

Building Trust Over Time

This book was designed to give you adaptability without turning you into a technician of your own body. You do not need to track everything. You do not need to supplement aggressively. You do not need to live in restriction. You need a clear framework and the confidence to trust it.

That confidence grows with experience. Each time you return to the blueprint and feel your body respond, trust builds. You learn what works for you specifically, not just what works in theory. You develop an instinct for when something is off and what might help. This instinct is not mysterious. It is pattern recognition built through repeated observation.

Trust also extends to the body itself. Many people have learned to distrust their bodies, treating them as problems to be managed rather than partners to be supported. The body's signals are dismissed as inconvenient. Its needs are seen as weaknesses. This adversarial relationship makes everything harder.

The blueprint invites a different relationship. The body is not broken. It knows how to clear, repair, and adapt. The role of the lifestyle is not to force these processes but to create conditions where they can happen naturally. When conditions are right, the body responds. Trust develops from seeing that response over and over again.

Detox becomes less about effort and more about stewardship: caring for a system that already knows how to restore balance when supported.

Setbacks and Returns

Life will throw challenges that disrupt even the most stable routine. Illness, travel, family crises, job changes, emotional upheaval. These are not failures of discipline. They are simply life. The question is not whether disruption will happen but how you respond when it does.

A program mentality treats disruption as failure. You fell off the wagon. You need to start over. The reset creates pressure, which creates stress, which makes recovery harder. Each disruption feels like going back to square one.

A blueprint mentality treats disruption as normal. You drifted from the pattern. Now you return. There is no wagon to fall off because there was never a moving vehicle in the first place. There is only a set of principles that support the body when applied. During disruption, application becomes partial. After disruption, application resumes more fully. No drama required.

The return itself builds strength. Each time you navigate a disruption and find your way back, you prove to yourself that recovery is possible. The blueprint becomes more familiar. The body remembers what balance feels like and gravitates toward it. Over time, deviations matter less because the center holds.

This is where the lifestyle becomes truly sustainable. Not because you never stray, but because straying no longer creates crisis. The foundation is strong enough to absorb occasional stress without crumbling.

The Role of This Book

As you move forward, remember that this blueprint is not meant to replace medical care, nor is it meant to compete with it. It is an educational framework that helps you understand how daily choices interact with the body's natural processes. Used alongside appropriate guidance, it can support informed decisions and steadier habits.

The information here is not prescriptive. It does not tell you exactly what to eat, how much to move, or which supplements to take. It explains principles so that you can make those decisions in a way that fits your life, your body, and your circumstances. Principles last. Prescriptions become outdated.

The next step after this book is not another detox challenge. It is application.

Application looks like small, repeated choices. Choosing meals that support stability. Choosing movement that encourages flow. Choosing rest without guilt. Choosing tools, whether herbs, supplements, or practices, only when they serve the foundation rather than distract from it.

Each choice is small. Together, they create the conditions for the body to do what it already knows how to do. That is the power of a lifestyle approach: nothing dramatic, everything cumulative.

When Detox Becomes Living

When detox becomes a way of living, health stops feeling fragile. Deviations matter less because recovery is built in. The body is not held together by constant intervention. It is supported by a rhythm that has become second nature.

You stop thinking about toxins and start thinking about how you want to feel. You stop counting days on a program and start noticing how the seasons of your life call for different kinds of support. You stop worrying about doing detox perfectly and start trusting that the body knows what to do when given half a chance.

This is the true outcome of the blueprint. Not a temporary cleanse, but a body that knows how to clear, recover, and adapt. A body that feels less mysterious because you understand how it works. A mind that feels less anxious because you know what to do when things drift off course.

And that is not a program you finish. It is a way of living you grow into.

The journey from here is yours. The blueprint provides direction. Experience provides wisdom. And the body, given the right conditions, provides the rest.

AFTERWORD

From Understanding to Mastery

If you have made it to the end of this book, you now understand something many people never stop to consider: detox is not a product, a program, or a moment in time. It is a biological process that either works quietly in the background or struggles under constant pressure.

This book was written to give you clarity.

You now understand how the body clears waste, how modern life interferes with that process, and how simple, repeatable choices can restore balance. You have learned why rhythm matters more than extremes, why support works better than force, and why detox becomes sustainable only when it fits into real life.

But understanding, on its own, is only the beginning.

Knowledge creates awareness. Mastery comes from application.

As you move forward, you may notice a natural next question forming: How do I put all of this together consistently, without guesswork? How do you translate principles into routines? How do you adjust for your lifestyle, your environment, your stress levels, and your season of life?

That is the purpose of *The Detox Mastery System.*

Where this book provides the framework, *The Detox Mastery System* provides the structure. It is a guided, video-first course designed to help you apply what you have learned here in a clear, organized, and practical way, without overwhelm.

The course is built as a self-paced experience, allowing you to move through the material at a rhythm that works for you. It combines core teaching with expert insight, practical demonstrations, and simple tools that help turn knowledge into daily habits. Rather than adding complexity, it is designed to remove it.

The Detox Mastery System is organized into four focused modules.

- The **first module** lays the foundation by revisiting detox as a biological system, not a trend. It walks through liver function, gut elimination, kidney and skin support, sleep and brain recovery, and how to recognize where detox is breaking down, without relying on guesswork or extremes. The goal is to help you see the body as a coordinated system and to reinforce the idea of detox as partnership, not punishment.

- The **second module** focuses on removing unnecessary load. Modern detox struggles are rarely caused by a single toxin. They are the result of constant, low-grade exposure, from food, water, and daily environments. This module helps you identify where that load actually comes from and how to reduce it through whole foods, hydration strategy, and simple environmental swaps. The emphasis is not perfection, but practicality.

- The **third module** moves into support. Modern life places demands on the body that traditional lifestyles did not. This is where herbs, roots, and supplements can be used responsibly. You will learn how ancestral tools align with modern biology, how to evaluate supplement quality, how to avoid dependency, and how timing and consistency matter more than quantity. Practical demonstrations show how to prepare teas, infusions, and simple remedies so these tools remain approachable rather than intimidating.

- The **final module** focuses on long-term living. Detox becomes sustainable only when it integrates into daily rhythm. This module addresses hydration, movement, sweat, lymph flow, sleep routines, stress reduction, and seasonal adjustments. It reframes detox as a lifestyle that builds resilience over time, so health feels less fragile and less reactive.

Throughout the course, you will also find downloadable worksheets and checklists designed to help you build routines without turning health into a full-time job. The goal is not constant intervention, but clarity and confidence.

Importantly, this course is not meant to replace this book. It expands it.

This book gives you the why. *The Detox Mastery System* gives you the how, the when, and the what if. It is for those who want guidance, structure, and demonstration, without losing the principles that keep detox grounded and sustainable.

You do not need to rush into the course. The blueprint you have learned here can already begin working in your life. But if you find yourself wanting deeper support, clearer routines, and a guided path toward long-term detox resilience, *The Detox Mastery System* exists for that reason.

Ultimately, the goal has never been to keep you detoxing.

The goal is to help you live in a way that does not require constant correction.

If this book has helped you see your body as capable rather than fragile, ordered rather than chaotic, and worthy of thoughtful care rather than constant force, then it has done its job.

Where you go next is up to you.

Whether you continue applying what you have learned on your own or choose to deepen that work through *The Detox Mastery System*, the most important step has already been taken: you have shifted from reacting to your health to understanding it.

And that shift changes everything!

The Detox Mastery System

The Complete Video Course

*"You now have the blueprint.
Are you ready for mastery?"*

INSIDE THE COURSE

✓ Step-by-step video modules that turn knowledge into daily practice

✓ Practical demonstrations for teas, infusions, and herbal preparation

✓ Downloadable worksheets and checklists for lasting habit change

✓ Interviews with Experts in Health & Nutrition

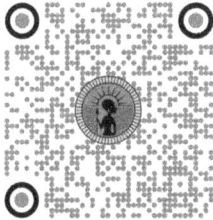

Scan to Enroll

Or visit the link below to learn more and continue your journey.

VISIT

www.ancientafricansecrets.com/detoxmastery

This book gave you the **why**.
The course gives you the **how**, the **when**,
and the **confidence** to make it last.

——— ◆ ———

REFERENCES

1. Anderson, J. W., & Konz, E. C. (2001). Obesity and disease management: Effects of weight loss on comorbid conditions. Obesity Research, 9(S11), 326S–334S.
2. Bachour, G., et al. (2025). Effects of Ashwagandha supplements on cortisol, stress, and anxiety levels in adults: A systematic review and meta-analysis. BJPsych Open, 11(2), e68.
3. Bischoff, S. C., et al. (2014). Intestinal permeability: A new target for disease prevention and therapy. BMC Gastroenterology, 14, 189.
4. Boden, G., Chen, X., & Urbain, J. L. (1996). Evidence for a circadian rhythm of insulin sensitivity in patients with NIDDM. Diabetes, 45(8), 1044–1050.
5. Ceriello, A., & Motz, E. (2004). Is oxidative stress the pathogenic mechanism underlying insulin resistance, diabetes, and cardiovascular disease? Arteriosclerosis, Thrombosis, and Vascular Biology, 24(5), 816–823.
6. Chaix, A., et al. (2014). Time-restricted feeding is a preventative and therapeutic intervention against diverse nutritional challenges. Cell Metabolism, 20(6), 991–1005.
7. Cherpak, C. E., & Freund, G. G. (2019). Mindful eating: A review of how the stress-digestion-mindfulness triad may modulate and improve gastrointestinal function. American Journal of Lifestyle Medicine, 14(2), 173–184.
8. Claus, S. P., Guillou, H., & Ellero-Simatos, S. (2016). The gut microbiota: A major player in the toxicity of environmental pollutants? NPJ Biofilms and Microbiomes, 2, 16003.
9. Cueni, L. N., & Detmar, M. (2008). The lymphatic system in health and disease. Lymphatic Research and Biology, 6(3–4), 109–122.
10. Deloose, E., et al. (2017). The migrating motor complex: Control mechanisms and its role in health and disease. Nature Reviews Gastroenterology & Hepatology, 9(5), 271–285.
11. DiNicolantonio, J. J., & O'Keefe, J. H. (2018). Omega-6 vegetable oils as a driver of coronary heart disease. Open Heart, 5(2), e000898.
12. Fan, M., et al. (2023). Dandelion (Taraxacum genus): A review of chemical constituents, pharmacological activities, and quality control. Frontiers in Pharmacology, 14, 1180840.
13. Feher, J. (2012). Quantitative Human Physiology: An Introduction (2nd ed.). Academic Press.
14. Finkel, T., & Holbrook, N. J. (2000). Oxidants, oxidative stress and the biology of ageing. Nature, 408(6809), 239–247.

15. Furman, D., et al. (2019). Chronic inflammation in the etiology of disease across the life span. Nature Medicine, 25, 1822–1832.
16. Gashev, A. A. (2008). Physiologic aspects of lymphatic contractile function. Annals of the New York Academy of Sciences, 1131, 100–109.
17. Grandjean, P., & Landrigan, P. J. (2014). Neurobehavioural effects of developmental toxicity. The Lancet Neurology, 13(3), 330–338.
18. Grant, D. M. (1991). Detoxification pathways in the liver. Journal of Inherited Metabolic Disease, 14(4), 421–430.
19. Häussinger, D. (1990). Nitrogen metabolism in liver: Structural and functional organization. Biochemical Journal, 267(2), 281–290.
20. Hodges, R. E., & Minich, D. M. (2015). Modulation of metabolic detoxification pathways using foods and food-derived components. Journal of Nutrition and Metabolism, 2015, 760689.
21. Hofmann, A. F. (1999). The continuing importance of bile acids in liver and intestinal disease. Archives of Internal Medicine, 159(22), 2647–2658.
22. Hu, F. B. (2002). Dietary pattern analysis: A new direction in nutritional epidemiology. Current Opinion in Lipidology, 13(1), 3–9.
23. Jensen, T., et al. (2018). Fructose and sugar: A major mediator of non-alcoholic fatty liver disease. Journal of Hepatology, 68(5), 1063–1075.
24. Kortenkamp, A. (2007). Ten years of mixing cocktails: A review of combination effects of endocrine-disrupting chemicals. Environmental Health Perspectives, 115(S1), 98–105.
25. Kuan, W.-H., Chen, Y.-L., & Liu, C.-L. (2022). Excretion of Ni, Pb, Cu, As, and Hg in sweat under two sweating conditions. Int. J. Environmental Research and Public Health, 19(7), 4323.
26. La Merrill, M., et al. (2013). Toxicological function of adipose tissue: Focus on persistent organic pollutants. Environmental Health Perspectives, 121(2), 162–169.
27. Landrigan, P. J., et al. (2018). The Lancet Commission on pollution and health. The Lancet, 391(10119), 462–512.
28. Lewis, S. J., & Heaton, K. W. (1997). Stool form scale as a useful guide to intestinal transit time. Scandinavian Journal of Gastroenterology, 32(9), 920–924.
29. Liska, D. J. (1998). The detoxification enzyme systems. Alternative Medicine Review, 3(3), 187–198.
30. Mayer, E. A., Tillisch, K., & Gupta, A. (2015). Gut/brain axis and the microbiota. Journal of Clinical Investigation, 125(3), 926–938.
31. McMullen, M. K., & Whitehouse, J. M. (2015). Bitters: Time for a new paradigm. Evidence-Based Complementary and Alternative Medicine, 2015, 670504.
32. Michalopoulos, G. K. (2007). Liver regeneration. Journal of Cellular Physiology, 213(2), 286–300.
33. Monteiro, C. A., et al. (2018). The UN Decade of Nutrition, the NOVA food classification and the trouble with ultra-processing. Public Health Nutrition, 21(1), 5–17.
34. Pareek, A., et al. (2023). Moringa oleifera: An updated comprehensive review of its pharmacological activity. Frontiers in Pharmacology, 14, 1110327.
35. Reinke, H., & Asher, G. (2019). Crosstalk between metabolism and circadian

clocks. Nature Reviews Molecular Cell Biology, 20(4), 227–241.

36. Ridlon, J. M., Kang, D. J., & Hylemon, P. B. (2006). Bile salt biotransformations by human intestinal bacteria. Journal of Lipid Research, 47(2), 241–259.

37. Salah, H. M., et al. (2022). Diaphragmatic function in cardiovascular disease. J. American College of Cardiology, 80(17), 1647–1659.

38. Samavat, H., & Kurzer, M. S. (2015). Estrogen metabolism and breast cancer. Cancer Letters, 356(2), 231–243.

39. Sears, M. E., Kerr, K. J., & Bray, R. I. (2012). Arsenic, cadmium, lead, and mercury in sweat: A systematic review. J. Environmental and Public Health, 2012, 184745.

40. Simopoulos, A. P. (2002). The importance of the ratio of omega-6/omega-3 essential fatty acids. Biomedicine & Pharmacotherapy, 56(8), 365–379.

41. Slavin, J. (2013). Fiber and prebiotics: Mechanisms and health benefits. Nutrients, 5(4), 1417–1435.

42. Spiegel, K., Leproult, R., & Van Cauter, E. (1999). Impact of sleep debt on metabolic and endocrine function. The Lancet, 354(9188), 1435–1439.

43. Sutton, E. F., et al. (2018). Early time-restricted feeding improves insulin sensitivity, blood pressure, and oxidative stress. Cell Metabolism, 27(6), 1212–1221.

44. Trefts, E., Gannon, M., & Wasserman, D. H. (2017). The liver. Current Biology, 27(21), R1147–R1151.

45. Uribarri, J., et al. (2010). Advanced glycation end products in foods and a practical guide to their reduction. J. American Dietetic Association, 110(6), 911–916.

46. Xie, L., et al. (2013). Sleep drives metabolite clearance from the adult brain. Science, 342(6156), 373–377.

47. Zanger, U. M., & Schwab, M. (2013). Cytochrome P450 enzymes in drug metabolism. Pharmacology & Therapeutics, 138(1), 103–141.

www.ingramcontent.com/pod-product-compliance
Lightning Source LLC
Chambersburg PA
CBHW030853270326
41928CB00008B/1349